PSYCHODYNAMICS OF DRUG DEPENDENCE

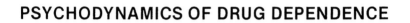

PSYCHODYNAMICS OF DRUG DEPENDENCE

Editors

Jack D. Blaine, M.D.
Demetrios A. Julius, M.D.

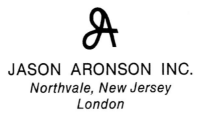

JASON ARONSON INC.
Northvale, New Jersey
London

Rc
564
·P79
1993

ACKNOWLEDGMENTS

Chapter 4, "Mr. Pecksniff's Horse? (Psychodynamics in Compulsive Drug Use)," by Leon Wurmser, is taken in slightly altered form from THE HIDDEN DIMENSION: PSYCHO-PATHOLOGY OF COMPULSIVE DRUG USE, published by Jason Aronson Inc. The appendix for Chapter 5 is reprinted with the permission of International Universities Press, Inc., from the *Journal of the American Psychoanalytic Association*, Vol. 21, No. 2, 1973.

THE MASTER WORK SERIES

DHEW publication number (ADM) 77-470, 1977.

Reprinted 1993

Library of Congress Cataloging-in-Publication Data *pending*

ISBN: 1-56821-157-0 (softcover)

Manufactured in the United States of America. Jason Aronson Inc. offers books and cassettes. For information and catalog write to Jason Aronson Inc., 230 Livingston Street, Northvale, New Jersey 07647.

PREFACE

The explanatory power of the new psychology of the self is no-where as evident as with regard to these four types of psychological disturbance: (1) the narcissistic personality disorders, (2) the perversions, (3) the delinquencies, and (4) the addictions. Why can these seemingly disparate conditions be examined so fruitfully with the aid of the same conceptual framework? Why can all these widely differing and even contrasting symptom pictures be comprehended when seen from the viewpoint of the psychology of the self? How, in other words, are these four conditions related to each other? What do they have in common, despite the fact that they exhibit widely differing, and even contrasting, symptomatologies? The answer to these questions is simple: in all of these disorders the afflicted individual suffers from a central weakness, from a weakness in the core of his personality. He suffers from the consequences of a defect in the self. The symptoms of these disorders, whether comparatively hazy or hidden, or whether more distinct and conspicuous, arise secondarily as an outgrowth of a defect in the self. The manifestations of these disorders become intelligible if we call to mind that they are all attempts—unsuccessful attempts, it must be stressed—to remedy the central defect in the personality.

The narcissistically disturbed individual yearns for praise and approval or for a merger with an idealized supportive other because he cannot sufficiently supply himself with self-approval or with a sense of strength through his own inner resources. The pervert is driven toward sexual enactments with figures or symbols that give him the feeling of being wanted, real, alive, or powerful. The delinquent repeats over and over again certain acts through which he demonstrates to himself an escape from the realization that he feels devoid of sustaining self-confidence and of sustaining ideals. And the addict, finally, craves the drug because the drug seems to him to be capable of curing the central defect in his self. It becomes for him the substitute for a self-object which failed him traumatically at a time when he should still have had the feeling of omnipotently controlling its responses in accordance with his needs as if it were a part of himself. By ingesting the drug he symbolically compels the mirroring self-object to soothe him, to accept him. Or he symbolically compels the idealized self-object to submit to his merging into it and thus to his partaking in its magical power. In either case the ingestion of the drug provides him with the self-esteem which he does not possess. Through the incorporation of the drug he supplies for himself the feeling of being accepted and thus of being self-confident; or he creates the experience of being merged with a source of power that gives him the feeling of being strong and worthwhile. And all these effects of the drug tend to increase his feeling of being alive, tend to increase his certainty that he exists in this world.

It is the tragedy of all these attempts at self-cure that the solutions which they provide are impermanent, that in essence they cannot succeed. The praise which the narcissistically disturbed individual is able to evoke, the mergers with idealized others which he brings about, the sexualized reassurances which the pervert procures for himself, the loudly proclaimed assertion of omnipotence forever repeated through his actions by the delinquent—they all give only fleeting relief. They are repeated again and again without producing the cure of the basic psychological malady. And the calming or the stimulating effect which the addict obtains from the drug is similarly impermanent. Whatever the chemical nature of the substance that is employed, however frequently repeated its consumption, however cleverly rationalized or mythologized its ingestion with the support from others who are similarly afflicted—no psychic structure is built, the defect in the self remains. It is as if a person with a wide open gastric fistula were trying to still his hunger through eating. He may obtain pleasurable taste sensations by his frantic ingestion of food but, since the food does not enter that part of the digestive system where it is absorbed into the organism, he continues to starve.

The enriching effect of the insights supplied by the psychology of the self upon the data obtained within different psychological frames of reference can be demonstrated with special clarity with regard to the examination of the family background, of the childhood situation of the future addict. It is evidently of great importance in the present context to determine certain details concerning the behavior of the addict's parents when he was a child. We might ask, for example, whether they had been lenient or strict, or whether their identities (e.g., as male and female; or, occupationally, the mother as a housewife, the father as a truckdriver, etc.) were hazy or well defined. Yet, having obtained the answer to these and similar questions, we will look at the significance of the socio-psychological data concerning parental behavior with different eyes when we examine them against the background of our knowledge concerning the factors that contribute to the child's ability to build up a strong and cohesive self and, in the obverse, concerning the factors that stand in the way of this crucial developmental task.

Just as we know, from the point of view of the physiologist, that a child needs to be given certain foods, that he needs to be protected against extreme temperatures, and that the atmosphere he breathes has to contain sufficient oxygen, if his body is to become strong and resilient, so do we also know, from the point of view of the depth-psychologist, that he requires an empathic environment— specifically, an environment that responds (a) to his need to have his presence confirmed by the glow of parental pleasure and (b) to his need to merge into the reassuring calmness of the powerful adult— if he is to acquire a firm and resilient self. It is not enough to obtain answers to questions such as whether the mother's attitude toward toilet training is strict or lenient, for example, or whether the father's work-identity is clearly defined or not. The crucial question concerns the adequacy or inadequacy of the parents as the self-objects of the child, i.e., the adequacy or inadequacy of the parents at a time when they are still performing for the child the psychological functions of self-esteem regulation which the child should later be able to perform on his own, the adequacy or inadequacy of the parents at a time in other words when the child still experiences them predominantly as extensions of himself or experiences himself still predominantly as part of their strength. The crucial question then is whether the parents are able to reflect with approval at least some of the child's proudly exhibited attributes and functions, whether they are able to respond with genuine enjoyment to his budding skills, whether they are able to remain in touch with him throughout his trials and errors. And, furthermore, we must determine whether they are able to provide the child with a reliable embodiment of calmness and strength into which he can merge and with a focus for his need to find a target for his admiration. Or, stated in the obverse, it will be of crucial importance to ascertain the fact that a child could find neither confirmation of his own worthwhileness nor a target for a merger with the idealized strength of the parent and that he, therefore, remained deprived of the opportunity for the gradual transformation of these external sources of narcissistic sustenance into endopsychic resources, i.e., specifically into sustaining self-esteem and into a sustaining relationship to internal ideals. Thus, in asking the crucial question concerning the factors in childhood which lead to the addiction-prone personality, we will say that, in the last analysis, and within certain limits, it is less important to determine what the parents *do* than what they *are*.

Heinz Kohut, M.D.
Institute for Psychoanalysis
Chicago

CONTENTS

CHAPTER 1

Introduction

Jack D. Blaine, M.D., and Demetrios A. Julius, M.D.

The Clinical-Behavioral Branch, Division of Research, NIDA, is interested in developing a comprehensive and practical approach to treatment of heroin-dependent people and drug abusers more generally. This approach should be based on a theoretically sound knowledge of the psychiatric status of the drug-dependent person as well as the psychodynamics of drug abuse and psychological dependence. The goal is to increase the quality of treatment and likelihood of successful therapeutic outcome by focusing on the individual's intrapsychic dynamics and relevant external factors, in order to select the most suitable treatment. Unfortunately, many gaps still exist in our knowledge about use, abuse, and dependence on opiates and other psychoactive drugs. One objective of this monograph is to stimulate the development of new research directions and strategies for implementing innovative treatment which take into consideration psychiatric evaluation and psychodynamic understanding.

With this in mind, the first Technical Review of the Psychodynamics of Drug Dependence convened on April 2 and 3, 1976, in Washington, D.C. Participants presented papers from which the substance of this monograph is primarily derived. To exploit the theoretical groundwork laid at this meeting, the technical review group recommended an ongoing series of small working groups, each of which would focus on a specific issue. Consequently, a second review group convened on March 17 and 18, 1977, to focus specifically on diagnostic and therapeutic research issues. The second group included some noted theoreticians and researchers in areas related to drug dependence, among them Harriet Barr, Otto Kernberg, Gerald Klerman, George Woody, Charles O'Brien, Catherine Treece and Henry Rosett, in addition to members of the first group

1

who continue active research in the area. We wish to thank all of these researchers and clinicians for the high caliber of interest and effort they have contributed.

The overview presented in chapter 2 was written before the second conference took place and therefore does not refer to it. We are, however, gratified to be able to include Dr. Woody's report as the final chapter of this monograph.

BACKGROUND

Before the early 1970's, an effort was made with each patient in drug abuse treatment to achieve an understanding of the specific personality structure and the psychodynamic factors contributing to the patient's drug dependence. This understanding formed the basis for therapeutic goals and course. Drug abuse treatment has historically utilized therapeutic communities, residential centers, outpatient drug-free treatment clinics, and detoxification clinics. These treatment modalities have used group therapy, psychopharmacological agents, individual counseling, family therapy and/or a therapeutic milieu as primary behavioral change-producing techniques.

The failure of heroin withdrawal alone as a treatment with the goal of long-term continued abstinence has been voluminously documented. At best, medically controlled detoxification had only immediate and temporary value as a first step in a comprehensive rehabilitation program. Medically regulated detoxification reduced human suffering and freed individuals from their physical dependence on heroin, which permitted a shift in attention to other more constructive pursuits. However, even long periods of confinement in a hospital, prison, or residential facility with traditional psychotherapeutic intervention have not significantly altered the subsequent relapse to heroin for the vast majority of addicts.

The advent of the methadone maintenance treatment modality and its large-scale application in the late sixties and early seventies in response to an epidemic increase in heroin addiction made dramatic alterations in the philosophy, process, and economics of heroin treatment. Methadone has proved to be an extremely effective pharmacologic agent. The drug is capable, when prescribed and taken properly, of providing symptomatic relief of the most apparent symptoms of heroin dependence: abstinence symptoms, craving, and blockade of euphoria resulting from opiate injection.

This medication can remove the need for using illicit heroin and potentially allows the individual to alter his deviant lifestyle. However, methadone alone does not alter the underlying psychopathology manifested in compulsive drug abuse and dependence or the unbearable feelings or fears that may trigger the compulsion. Methadone maintenance is in many ways analogous to the use of phenothiazines in the treatment of schizophrenia. The phenothiazines have dramatic effect on the psychotic manifestations of decompensated schizophrenics, facilitating long-term psychotherapy and rehabilitation, which are important treatment components.

The availability of an effective symptomatic treatment modality, coupled with rapid expansion of the heroin-dependent population, produced an increased demand for treatment. As a result, treatment resources did not keep pace with the increased demand for treatment, producing waiting lists, expanded patient case loads, utilization of paraprofessional counselors, and an emphasis on cost-effective treatment. All these factors contributed to a shift in treatment emphasis from intrapsychic factors to external social and economic aspects of the client's life. Goals of treatment also concomitantly shifted from basic personality growth and comprehensive personal rehabilitation to social rehabilitation or merely changing social behaviors. Evaluation of outcome focused on lifestyle (e.g., use of illicit drugs and alcohol abuse, illegal activity, general health, arrests) and social productivity (e.g., employment, educational achievements, marital stability).

Despite the substantiated positive effect methadone maintenance has had for many thousands of heroin-dependent individuals on social rehabilitation, the ability to become and remain drug free after treatment has again become a criterion of success for many of those who articulate drug policy. However, relatively little effort has been made to understand or treat the psychopathology which contributes to the individual's psychological dependence on heroin and prevents meeting that criterion.

Recently, there has been renewed interest in developing a deeper comprehension of the psychodynamics of drug dependence in the light of recent advances in psychoanalytic ego theory. Much of this interest has been generated by accounts of the thoughtful and provocative clinical work of the psychoanalytic clinicians represented in this monograph working with drug-abusing populations. These clinicians have proposed major theoretical advances toward achieving an understanding of drug abuse and psychological dependence. Many have extended this theoretical framework to propose implications for psychotherapy and treatment of drug abuse and especially psychological drug dependence. These contributions, as well as those of others represented in the bibliography, are discussed in the following paper by Khantzian and Treece.

DIAGNOSIS

A central issue in evaluating different treatment methods for
drug abuse has been increasing dissatisfaction with the uncritical
acceptance of "drug abuse" as a diagnostically homogeneous term.
Both the clinical and research literature look generically at the
effects of treatment on drug abusers, and only rarely has a clinician
or scientist attempted to develop a treatment directed at a more
specific diagnostic entity.

Reemphasis on psychiatric diagnosis implicitly reflects a conviction that "drug abuse" is not a genuine diagnostic entity. Rather, it
is an attempt to categorize people in terms of an overt behavior
which may express several genuine diagnostic entities and which
may at times probably exist in the absence of psychopathology.
Yet it is difficult to see how treatment can be efficacious, especially
for long-term, rehabilitative goals, so long as we continue to treat
individuals having different psychopathologies with a hodge-podge
of treatments specific to none of them.

Some may question whether the specialty of psychiatry currently
possesses the technology for specific psychiatric diagnosis. It is true
that diagnostic classification in psychiatry is in the process of
development and refinement in an attempt to integrate new information and perspectives generated by different schools of theoretical orientation, e.g., psychoanalytic ego psychology and biological
psychiatry.

The 1968 edition of *Diagnostic and Statistical Manual of Mental
Disorders* (DSM-II) prepared by the American Psychiatric Association represents an attempt to achieve this goal. The APA is currently developing a DSM-III to reflect changes in the field. Concur-
rently, each of the different schools of thought in psychiatry is
clarifying the field from its own unique perspective. As a result, the
scientific literature and popular press abound with a variety of diagnostic nomenclatures for psychiatric patients in general and drug
users and abusers in particular. However, this dynamic state of the
art and science of psychiatry should not be viewed as a limiting
factor. In fact, psychiatry has been undergoing change since its
inception. Generally, this process has resulted in advancement for
psychiatry as a medical specialty and better treatment for patients
having psychiatric illnesses. Thus, focusing the attention of psychiatric diagnosticians and innovative clinicians on the often-over-
looked population of drug abusers has potential benefit for psychiatry as well as afflicted individuals.

DSM-II includes the category "drug dependence" (304) ". . . for
patients who are addicted to or dependent on drugs other than

alcohol, tobacco, and ordinary caffeine-containing beverages, and unindicated or inappropriately taken prescribed drugs. The diagnosis requires evidence of habitual use or a clear sense of need for the drug. The diagnosis may stand alone or be coupled with any other diagnosis" (DSM-II, 1968, p. 45).

Indeed, the psychiatric diagnoses of "sociopathic personality disorder" and "psychopathic personality disorder" have been used by some writers in this field in the past, supposedly to clarify what and who a "drug abuser" is. However, this type of diagnostic effort has merely led to the widespread feeling that these diagnostic labels are no more clarifying than the descriptive label "drug abuser" itself. In fact, these diagnostic categories have now disappeared from the official American Psychiatric Association's Diagnostic and Statistical Manual of Mental Disorders (DSM-II), and have been replaced by the term "antisocial personality" (301.7). The official definition reads, in part, "This term is reserved for individuals who are basically unsocialized and whose behavior pattern brings them repeatedly into conflict with society. They are incapable of significant loyalty to individuals, groups, or social values. They are grossly selfish, callous, irresponsible, impulsive, and unable to feel guilt or to learn from experience and punishment . . ." (DSM-II, 1968, p. 43). Although this may characterize some drug-dependent individuals, it does not characterize the vast majority. The language of this diagnostic category implies, in effect, that such people are unfit to interrelate with "normal" people and should be seen as a deviant subgroup for whom there is probably little help possible.

Applying this type of diagnosis to the drug-dependent person is of little practical value. What is necessary for practical treatment is either to identify other major, treatable components of these individuals' psychic constellation or to more explicitly and completely diagnose (Gr., *dia* — through, between; *gignoskein* — to know) what we now call antisocial personality and other applicable subdiagnoses. With regard to the first necessity, researchers have, for example, begun to demonstrate the existence of a subgroup of dependent individuals who can be diagnosed as depressed.

In an unpublished report, Senay (1975) has demonstrated the existence of significant depressive symptomatology in a group of opiate users in Chicago. Weissman, et al. (1976) have also demonstrated the same result. Using standard rating scales of depression, they have shown that a substantial minority of methadone-maintained patients are, in fact, clinically depressed. The implications of such results, of course, lead to a refinement of treatment plans for such patients. In this regard, the double-blind placebo-controlled pilot study of Woody, O'Brien, and Rickels (1975) has shown a significant improvement of methadone maintenance patients who received the antidepressant agent, doxepin, over those who received the placebo. However, this was only a preliminary study, and longer term studies utilizing similar designs are now underway to validate these results. When these studies are completed, they may shed light on which type of treatment is most effective for this subgroup of drug-dependent individuals.

From this exemplary exploration of a new diagnostic area we see that there is indeed diagnostic thinking already available to identify one subgroup of drug users. This thinking also has direct implications for treatment of these individuals. Diagnoses within the general category of "depression" are also continually being refined. Psychopharmacologists have identified syndromes of retarded depressions, agitated depressions, hostile depressions, reactive depressions, and endogenous depressions. What is of value in this subclassification is that each of these subgroups seems to do better within certain specific treatment regimens. For example, Gershon, Hekimian, and Floyd (1967) have shown, in a placebo-controlled study, that 70 to 80 percent of patients with retarded depressions do best with the tricyclic antidepressants. Hollister and Overall (1965) have also lent supporting evidence for this treatment, in that they found this group of depressions to respond best to imipramine (a tricyclic antidepressant), while thioridazine (a phenothiazine) was of little value. However, in hostile depressions, the same study found thioridazine and imipramine to be equally effective. And in the reactive depressions, if the patient is receptive to verbal therapy, psychoanalytically oriented psychotherapy produces equally effective, if not superior, results to chemotherapy. Other schools of theoretical orientation may view depression differently, resulting in other diagnostic terminology, e.g., primary and secondary affective disorder or manic-depressive disease. Nevertheless, the foregoing and other studies have shown how more specific differential diagnoses can improve treatment regimens with correspondingly enhanced chances for successful outcomes.

Returning to the more difficult classification of character or personality disorder such as sociopathic, psychopathic, antisocial, narcissistic, and borderline personality disorders, how can we proceed in the same fashion as we have shown is possible in the classification of depression? Part of the answer may lie within recent advances in psychoanalytic thinking. The work of Greenacre, Kohut, and Kernberg has deepened and expanded the understanding of character pathology in general, and the so-called borderline and narcissistic personality disorders in particular. This pioneering work, drawing on solid observational and treatment interaction data, is evolving a complex and sophisticated theoretical base upon which can be built further concrete understanding of an enigmatic region of personality pathology. There is, however, a need to distill and condense much of this thinking down to identifiable subgroups, which then would have specific implications for specific treatment regimens. In applying these new theoretical insights to the diagnostic problem of "drug abusers," as well as developing new theoretical avenues of their own, researchers such as Khantzian, Wurmser, Krystal, Frosch, Wieder, and Kaplan have all begun the work of distillation of the theoretical work already accomplished. Their work is now leading to more practical, specific, and operational formulations of diagnosis and consequent treatment planning of drug-dependent individuals.

The process of arriving at operational diagnostic subcategories, therefore, moves from the more generic to descriptive categories sufficiently refined to indicate actual treatment. Diagnostically, we proceed from general descriptive terms such as "drug abuser" to more refined descriptors that indicate demographic variables. These include race, socioeconomic status, criminality, exposure to drugs, ethnic background and social environment, among others. These factors aid in understanding drug-dependent individuals, but do not in themselves dictate a complete treatment regimen. Further refinement leads to more specific diagnostic categories such as those found in the APA's DSM-II. These diagnoses include subgroups such as depressive neurosis, psychotic depression reaction, manic-depressive illness, or those with descriptive personality disorders. Categorization can stop at this point or proceed to further refinement, as we have seen in the subgroupings of depression. We advocate further refinement of the psychiatric diagnoses of the DSM-II. This refinement may be especially critical within the category of the antisocial, borderline personality. Within this subgroup we can begin to look at measures of such personality components as reality testing, structure of defense mechanisms, intactness of ego and super-ego functions, degree of grandiosity, identity diffusion, quality of object relations, and control of affects.

Can we, in fact, begin to define subgroups of individuals on the continuum of character pathology predominantly characterized by defects in one or more of these personality categories? To do so could have significant implications for differentiating treatment approaches. This process of refinement and exploration into undefined areas of personality diagnosis is undertaken by the contributors to this monograph.

TREATMENT

Improved psychiatric diagnosis in the field of drug abuse has at least four implications for treatment. The first and most immediately apparent is that patients could, when indicated, receive individual psychotherapy, group therapy, family therapy, or psychopharmacologic agents directed at their psychopathology, such as those already indicated for treatment of depression. This would occur in addition to opiate maintenance therapy, vocational training, and the like, directed at their chronic behavior disorder and social circumstances.

Evolving sophistication in diagnosis of drug-abusing individuals will have implications for those who are evaluating and treating these people. These developments will increase the demand on therapists to be more interested in, to show greater understanding of, and to have deeper empathy for the people they are helping. Specificity in diagnosis will also mean specificity in treatment. This should then lead to clinic treatment centers where multimodality approaches allow a wide range of treatment regimens for a wide range of subgroups of "drug abusers."

Currently, in many treatment programs the major responsibility for the assessment of psychological needs and provision of psychological treatment is given to paraprofessionals who are not trained in psychiatric diagnosis and treatment. Unfortunately, these well-intentioned counselors are not able to make use of the potentially valuable information available to them in planning and providing treatment services. Thus, the increased participation of psychiatrists in treatment clinics may provide training opportunities and supervision for paraprofessionals.

A more subtle implication would be the impact on the clinic as a treatment milieu. Currently, methadone clinics, for example, are generally structured according to the personal whim of their director or dominant staff members. They can be confronting or lax, can be structured or allow patients great latitude, can be only dispensaries or very active in their patients' lives. These different clinical structures have radically different implications for different personality types and for different psychopathologies. The way a clinic interacts with a patient can mean the difference between success or failure in initiating and keeping the patient in treatment. Similarly, the way a clinic is structured is important for the success it will have with different types of psychopathology. For example, with the borderline personality, the need to provide sufficient external structure is felt to be a precondition for treatment. The role and effect of methadone, residential communities, behavioral therapy, or clinic regulations in providing this need are yet to be determined. Hence, diagnosis is a necessary condition for providing a clinic milieu that will enhance treatment.

Finally, increasing our awareness of the types of psychopathology found in the drug abuse population will also increase our awareness of the psychotropic effects of drugs of abuse. For example, it is possible that heroin may have a beneficial effect on some individuals and may even constitute a form of self-medication. But our current lack of diagnostic specificity hinders understanding the function of abuse drugs in the psychopathology of our patients. It also hinders the exploration of when and how to replace abused drugs in those patients for whom the drug may serve a useful function.

CONCLUSION

Our awareness of the importance of diagnosis in drug abuse is only now emerging. Some of the relevant research questions raised are: Are there sufficient theoretical positions currently available to generate testable hypotheses for diagnosis and treatment? Is there a need to develop a more cohesive theory of the psychopathology and psychodynamics of compulsive abuse and psychological dependence? Do the manifested symptoms of compulsive abuse and psychological dependence (for example, narcotic hunger or craving, abstinence, euphoria) reflect structural defects of symbolic defense mechanisms? Is there benefit to be gained from availability of comprehensive psychotherapies in treatment programs? Can more effective treatment approaches be devised utilizing current knowledge? What are the implications for maintenance drug therapy or use of other psychopharmacologic agents? What are the implications for length and course of treatment? Would continued treatment of the patient after the symptom of drug dependence disappeared be beneficial, as in other chronic relapsing disorders with cycles of remission and exacerbation? What operational formulations can be developed for clinical testing?

There are also questions that relate to the psychopharmacology of opiates and other abused drugs: Are there specific psychotropic effects of opiates which are psychotherapeutic for the individual user? Do these effects differ for users with varying types and degress of psychopathology? What is the nature of these actions? Do they help bolster underdeveloped defense mechanisms necessary to master tensions and anxieties of daily life problems or intrapsychic conflicts?

The focus of this monograph on the illicit abused drugs, the opiates in particular, represents only a small proportion of abuse substances and habitual behaviors leading to a variety of difficulties for man. However, the abuse of illicit drugs may be viewed as the most deviant habitual behavior on a continuum which includes excessive use of alcohol, tobacco, and food. Perhaps a more complete understanding of the more deviant behavior will shed light on the more common but frequently self-destructive behaviors. The Division of Research, NIDA, hopes to stimulate definitive research in these areas. By encouraging well-conceptualized, well-designed research protocols, which are also placebo-controlled and double-blinded when necessary, we hope to provide convincing answers to these complex questions for researchers and therapists alike.

The papers presented in this monograph are an initial effort addressed to some of these questions by a group of psychiatrists, most of whom have had considerable experience with patients who are drug abusers and consequently have developed some feeling for the complexity of these questions. The papers range from the theoretical to the clinical and from broad-scope issues to quite precise, limited studies. Collectively, they give a flavor of the current state of the art.

REFERENCES

Diagnostic and Statistical Manual of Mental Disorders (DSM-II). Washington, D.C.: American Psychiatric Association, 1968, p. 43.

Gershon, S., Hekimian, L.J., and Floyd, A. Pre-clinical-clinical correlation of antidepressant activity: Controlled study of gamfexine and imipramine, *Curr Ther Res*, 9:349-354, 1967.

Hollister, L.E., and Overall, J.E. Reflections on the specificity of action of antidepressants. *Psychosomatics*, 6:361-365, 1965.

Overall, J.E., Hollister, L.E., Meyer, F., Kimbell, I., and Shelton, J. Imipramine and thioridazine in depressed and schizophrenic patients. Are these specific antidepressant drugs? *JAMA*, 189:605-608, 1964.

Senay, E. *Depression in Drug Abusers*. Chicago, University of Chicago, 1975 (unpublished report).

Weissman, M., Slobetz, F., Prusoff, B., Mezritz, M., and Howard, P. Clinical depression among narcotic addicts maintained on methadone in the community, *Am J Psychiatry*, 133(12):1434-1438, December 1976.

Woody, G., O'Brien, C., and Rickels, K. Depression and anxiety in heroin addicts: A placebo-controlled study of doxepin in combination with methadone, *Am J Psychiatry*, 132(4):447-450, April 1975.

CHAPTER 2

Psychodynamics of Drug Dependence: An Overview

Edward J. Khantzian, M.D., and Catherine J. Treece, Ph.D.

BACKGROUND

Until recently, attempts to apply psychoanalytic theory to an understanding and treatment of drug dependence have been limited, and when attempted, have proven inconsequential. Self-help and methadone maintenance approaches, which developed and proliferated in the 1960's, provided the mainstay of treatment for compulsive and chronic drug use. The promise that these two new modalities seemed to offer, corresponding with rising alarm about a drug problem in this country of "epidemic proportions," resulted in the development and expenditure of enormous resources at the Federal, State, and local levels to enlist large numbers of patients in treatment and rehabilitation. Unfortunately, the hope that vast expenditures would result in speedy cures and expeditiously eliminate the problem has proven illusory. The development of this monograph represents a modest but significant departure from these recent trends. In April of 1976, the Division of Research, Clinical-Behavioral Branch, under the leadership of Drs. Pollin, Renault, Julius and Blaine convened a group of psychoanalysts, psychiatrists and psychologists who had demonstrated an interest in understanding substance use from a psychodynamic point of view. The participants were charged to reexamine psychoanalytic theory and its relevance for understanding opiate addiction. There was also an implied hope that some practical treatment applications could be garnered from such an exercise.

The preliminary results of this effort are represented by the content of this monograph. We believe it represents a good beginning. With the interest and support of NIDA, the participants of and contributors to the first Technical Review in 1976 and to this monograph, have, in our estimation, demonstrated the value and utility of developing and expanding on previous applications of psychoanalytic theory to problems of substance use.

The study of addiction as a human process begs for a depth psychology. We are convinced that psychoanalytic theory continues to be the most enabling and useful depth psychology at our disposal to understand the human mind and behavior, including addictive behavior. Psychoanalysis does not invalidate other psychological methods of understanding, but rather attempts to account more adequately for the complexities of human behavior in terms of dynamic, economic, structural, developmental and adaptational factors. For the unversed in psychoanalytic theory the contents of this monograph might seem too complex, obscure and far removed from an everyday understanding and management of drug-dependent individuals. We believe that the theoretical formulations developed in this monograph reflect rather than obscure the complexities of the drug problems with which we work. We also believe that diligence in trying to comprehend this theoretical point of view will help to organize clinical observations and apply them more meaningfully and consistently in work with patients. In turn, hopefully, our theory will more likely reflect data and observations obtained from what our patients tell us and what they experience. Clearly, the clinical observations about drug-dependent patients and the theoretical discussions in this monograph suggest a number of avenues for further exploration and research. We believe that this beginning effort to involve psychoanalysts in national efforts to address problems of opiate addiction represents a promising vista for the development of a more dynamic clinical approach and a richer theoretical understanding of drug dependence.

The intention of this chapter is to provide an updated review of the literature and to provide an overview of this monograph, stressing areas of agreement and complementarity, as well as unresolved differences, among the contributors.

THE LITERATURE — AN UPDATE

Yorke (1970) and Khantzian (1974) have recently reviewed the early psychoanalytic literature on addiction. They have both concluded that the limitations of an excessively drive-oriented model prevented these early authors from fully developing and utilizing many important clinical observations. Thus, there was an excessive emphasis on the libidinal gratification provided through drug use to account for the addict's involvement with his drug. Similarly, in their overemphasis on the symbolic meaning of the drug and how it was used, they failed to make distinctions between various classes of drugs and their distinctive psychopharmacologic effects. Khantzian notes that Rado (1933, 1957), in particular, and Savit (1954), Fenichel (1945) and others, seemed to appreciate underlying depression and tension as motives for taking drugs. However, in his review Khantzian concludes that these themes are not well developed and that too much emphasis is placed on pleasurable and regressive aspects of drug use to explain the compelling nature of addiction. Although Glover (1956) also failed to appreciate the specific effects of different drugs and excessively stressed symbolic factors, Yorke and Khantzian have both noted that he better appreciated the adaptive, "progressive" use of drugs to cope with and defend against powerful, overwhelming and psychoticogenic rage and aggression.

The work of Chein et al. (1964) and the previous related work by Gerard and Kornetsky (1954) marks a significant shift in the psychoanalytic literature. Studying adolescent addiction in the ghetto rather than adult addiction in the analytic office provided new perspectives on which to build. In addition to appreciating the specific psychotropic effects of opiates, their work more adequately focused on the addict's ego and superego pathology, problems with narcissism and other psychopathology. They delineated some of the major difficulties that addicts have in engaging their environment, and stressed how their use of heroin was "adaptive and functional," helping them to overcome crippling adolescent anxieties evoked by the prospect of facing adult role expectations with inadequate preparation, models, and prospects. Subsequently, Hartmann (1969) developed similar themes through the study of other populations of adolescent drug users, focusing on the use of drugs, particularly by those with passive tendencies, to avoid active mastery of adolescent tasks in which narcotics were used to provide a passive regressive solution to intra-psychic conflicts associated with the adolescent phase of development. Wieder and Kaplan (1969) elaborated further on this point of view, emphasizing that preadolescent developmental conflicts left certain individuals specifically vulnerable to problems of anxiety, depression, and physical discomfort during adolescence. In such cases drugs seemed to provide the means to induce a desirable ego regression. Specific drugs were understood to be related to stage-specific developmental conflict. Opiates, for instance, were said to produce a state reminiscent of a blissful closeness and union with the mother, which resulted in avoidance of separation anxieties aroused by the adolescent dependency crisis.

Despite a superficial resemblance to earlier formulations that stressed regressive pleasurable use of drugs, their work represents an important advance and elaboration of trends set in motion by Gerard and Kornetsky in the 1950's which utilized recent developments in ego theory enabling Wieder and Kaplan to appreciate that individuals self-select different drugs based on personality organization and ego impairments. Their emphasis on the use of drugs as a "prosthetic," and their focus on developmental considerations, adaptation and the ego, clearly sets their work apart from earlier simplistic formulations based on an id psychology.

Based on this and other recent work that considers ego and adaptational problems of addicts and following lines pursued by Wieder and Kaplan, Milkman and Frosch (1973) empirically tested the hypothesis that self-selection of specific drugs is related to preferred defensive style. Using the Bellak and Hurvich Interview and Rating Scale for Ego Functioning, they compared heroin and amphetamine addicts in drugged and non-drugged conditions. Their preliminary findings supported their hypothesis that heroin addicts preferred the calming and dampening effects of opiates and seemed to use this action of the drug to shore up tenuous defenses and reinforce a tendency toward withdrawal and isolation, while amphetamine users used the stimulating action of amphetamines to support an inflated sense of self-worth and a defensive style involving active confrontation with their environment. Similarly, Hendin (1974), using psychological testing and interview data, concluded that heroin as well as barbiturates acted to assist in withdrawal and to avoid intimacy and thus defend against overwhelming destructive impulses.

In contradistinction, the works of Wurmser (1972, 1974) and Khantzian (1972, 1974, 1975) suggest that the excessive emphasis on the regressive effects of narcotics in these studies is unwarranted, and that in fact, the specific psychopharmacologic action of opiates has an opposite, "progressive" effect whereby regressed states may be reversed. Wurmser believes that narcotics are used adaptively by narcotic addicts to compensate for defects in affect defense, particularly against feelings of "rage, hurt, shame—and loneliness." Khantzian stresses drive defense and believes narcotics act to reverse regressed states by the direct antiaggression action of opiates, counteracting disorganizing influences of rage and aggression on the ego. Both these formulations propose that the psychopharmacologic effects of the drug can substitute for defective or non-existent ego mechanisms of defense. As with previously mentioned recent investigators, Wurmser and Khantzian also consider developmental impairments, the severe, predisposing psychopathology, and problems in adaptation as central issues in understanding addiction.

Radford, Wiseberg, and Yorke (1972) reported detailed case material that supports the findings of Wurmser and Khantzian that opiates can have an antiaggression and antiregression action or effect. They further observe that opiate use cannot be exclusively correlated with any particular patterns of internal conflict or phase-specific developmental impairment.

Despite differences in emphasis, the work of Gerard and Kornetsky, Hartmann, Wieder and Kaplan, Milkman and Frosch, and Hendin shares in common a stress on opiate use as an attempt to correct impaired or defective ego functions and thereby assist the individual to cope. It is also recurrently evident in the work of these investigators that this attempt is only partially successful at best. Their findings repeatedly seem to suggest that adopting passive solutions through opiates induces a self-perpetuating tendency for maladaptive and pathologic ego and drive regression. This apparent contradiction between the adaptive and maladaptive effects of opiate use implied in these formulations awaits further clarification.

Krystal and Raskin (1970) are somewhat less precise about the specific effects of different drugs, but allow that they may be used either to permit or prevent regression. However, their work does focus much more precisely on the relationship between the affects of pain, depression, and anxiety, and drug and placebo effects. Addicts' difficulties in recognizing and tolerating painful affects are explored and greatly clarified. The tendency for the affects of depression and anxiety to remain somatized, unverbalized and undifferentiated in addicts, results in a defective stimulus barrier and thus leaves such individuals ill-equipped to deal with their feelings, and predisposes them to drug use. Their work also focuses in greater depth on the major problems that addicts have in relation to positive and negative feelings about themselves and in relation to other people. Krystal and Raskin believe that addicts have major difficulties in being good to themselves and in dealing with their positive and negative feelings toward others because of rigid and massive defenses such as splitting and denial. They maintain that drug users take drugs not only to assist in defending against their feelings, but also briefly and therefore "safely" to enable the experience of feelings like fusion (oneness) with loved objects, which are normally prevented by the rigid defenses against aggression.

The problem of ego regression among narcotic addicts has been addressed by Zinberg (1975) from a rather different perspective than most of the other authors cited here. Zinberg minimizes factors of psychopathology and proposes an alternative explanation for the uniformly regressed appearance and behavior of addicts. Zinberg develops his thesis around the concept of relative autonomy of the ego. He suggests that the enforced social isolation and deviant status of illicit narcotics users result in a sufficient reduction of balanced input from external reality as to undermine the ego's relative autonomy from the id, and simultaneously affect superego structures which are maintained by social supports. The cyclical nature of addiction in which the user continuously cycles from high to low and back again serves to keep drive tension high which results in increased dependence on the environment for obtaining drugs and for whatever is left of coherent social relations, thus weakening relative autonomy from the environment. Under such conditions, Zinberg notes, the ego could be expected to undergo a regressive process resulting in the "typical impulse-ridden, psychopathic junkie" who is the subject of most clinical studies.

SUMMARY AND OVERVIEW OF THE MONOGRAPH

Dr. Wieder's paper begins the series of papers in this monograph with a proposal that we proceed from an historical perspective. He takes us back to an early period at Lexington where Federal efforts were first made to unravel the enigma of addiction and drug dependence through collaborative efforts of behavioral and biological scientists and psychiatrists. He recounts his experience as a member of these pioneering researchers, noting their difficulties even then in unifying a body of knowledge generated by researchers and clinicians who had yet to agree upon basic definitions of the phenomenon, the nature of the problem, or the constructs to be used in their study. Dr. Wieder reminds us of the interdependency of theory and data in scientific investigation, and challenges the technical review group to learn from what has gone before them. Before generating yet more voluminous data, he pleads for systematic evaluation of what has already been studied and learned. Wieder observes that despite the accumulation of massive, valuable data at Lexington, they were unable to develop a valid psychological definition or theory of addiction because of a restrictive medical model that was prevalent. Psychoanalysis was similarly unequal to the challenge as a result of its own definitional problems, wherein addiction was too narrowly defined as "an impulse problem" and therefore not within the domain of psychoanalysis. Because of exclusion of addicts from treatment based on inadequacies of earlier theory, plus the low socioeconomic background of most opiate addicts, few such patients were seen by analysts. Based on these trends, Wieder laments that the Lexington experience suffered from an absence of analysts, and that when analysts attempted to formulate an understanding of addiction, their formulation suffered because of an absence of comprehensive, objective clinical data. Wieder believes that Rado made a good beginning and that his insight, "not the toxic agent, but the impulse to use it," could have been an important cornerstone for a psychoanalytic theory of addiction. Wieder is skeptical that the application of any particular formulation by itself will greatly improve our treatment capabilities; however, he is firm in his conviction that psychoanalysis represents the most meaningful method of understanding human behavior and development, and applied to addiction, will make its greatest contributions in the areas of formulating and understanding the problem and in theory development.

The next four papers plunge directly into the rich complexity of psychoanalytic formulation. These papers exemplify the fact that psychoanalysis is not one theory, but many part theories, each addressing a different metapsychological level or a different explanatory perspective. This will be demanding reading for non-psychoanalytic readers, but well worth their while. As Dr. Wieder notes in closing, reminding us of the mandate of our work and the promise that it brings to this diverse field, psychoanalytic theory is the "most comprehensive view of human behavior" currently available.

Dr. Wurmser begins by reminding us of the importance of appreciating the severe psychopathology in compulsive drug users. He cautions the reader against the impulse to seek simple or expedient solutions to an immensely complex problem. In elaborating and expanding upon his own earlier observations (1974), Dr. Wurmser challenges us greatly to apply already complex concepts of narcissism, affect defense, compulsivity, splitting, psychological boundaries, and externalization to the analysis and understanding of the etiology of compulsive drug use. However, in pursuing the challenge and complexity of Wurmser's thinking, new and enriching vistas of understanding as well as valuable hints as to where we should be looking further are opened up for us. His meticulously developed model for what he considers the direct and specific psychological antecedents of compulsive drug use is an object lesson in the rewards of patience and perseverance in the face of such complexity. In this paper the knowledgeable clinician will find many occasions to nod his or her head in recognition as Dr. Wurmser unravels the threads of behavior and motivation, and puts them into a model which manages to allow for specific application within the framework of highly abstract concepts. And by reconsidering compulsive drug use in the light of more recent conceptual developments in psychoanalytic theory, Dr. Wurmser enriches and contemporizes both the drug field and the theories themselves.

Dr. Greenspan in his paper focuses primarily on the developmental and adaptational perspective within a psychoanalytic model of learning. He summarizes the major developmental challenges of early life, starting with the earliest phases of achieving homeostasis and need satisfying attachment, through subsequent phases of separation, individuation and capacity for mental representation (as developed by Mahler and Piaget). He stresses how optimal nurturance and encouragement from the environment (as primarily represented by the mother) fosters adequate mastery of these phases by the infant, and leads to the development of stable ego structures and capacities to manage drives and object relations. To the extent that the individual is overly deprived or indulged in his/her development, varying degrees of ego impairment occur and drugs then come to substitute and compensate for the developmental defects and impairments. Greenspan specifically delineates how the lack of integrated ego structures and differentiated drive organization in certain individuals leave them particularly susceptible to environmental reinforcers and influences. In the case of addicts, drugs as well as many other environmental influences become powerful determinants of behavior in the absence of adequate ego structures and drive organization. Notwithstanding a difference in terminology, this formulation is consistent with and bears important resemblance to Krystal's notions of developmental impairments in the stimulus barrier and the failure in differentiation of affects. It also parallels Wurmser's thinking, wherein he emphasizes the addict's need to externalize and to act in the absence of adequate ego defenses.

In the next paper, Krystal clarifies the defensive function of the "splitting" mechanism in drug-dependent individuals, and traces the enormous problems that addicts have with ambivalence, particularly aggression. He discusses the nature of childhood trauma which can lead to undifferentiated or regressed affects and poor affect tolerance. Such trauma, in later life, may result in a massive "walling off" of self- and object-representations and an inability to provide comforting and self-care maternal modes for the self, or to tolerate aggression toward significant objects. Krystal cogently describes the viscissitudes of these trends in the transference when long-term psychotherapy is undertaken with such patients. The work of therapy centers on helping the individual to overcome the fear of closeness with the therapist (i.e., vis-a-vis rekindled childhood longings and fears of aggressive impulses), learning to grieve effectively, owning up to one's destructive feelings, and finally, overcoming the barriers that prevent effective comforting and care of oneself. Krystal suggests that success in this process invalidates the need for the placebo and pharmacologic action of the drug to effect access to these parts and functions of the self.

Dr. Khantzian's paper serves to provide some perspective on what has gone before, by reviewing and pulling together the major themes embodied in the foregoing papers and in other recent literature. He then explores aspects of ego function related to drive defense and "self-care." He proposes a gap and/or impairment in the ego function of self-care. He relates this to failures in internalization of vital functions which have left the individual vulnerable to a whole range of hazardous behavior and involvement, but in particular, to addiction. He then goes on to review how certain narcissistic processes and resultant defenses are related to unique characteristics and traits of addicts that impair such individuals in obtaining satisfaction in their involvement with people, work and play.

The next three papers offer a sampling of clinical case material and research which follows from the preceding formulations. Dr. Davidson's paper brings a psychoanalytic understanding to an evaluation of methadone maintenance clinics as a treatment modality. She has provided valuable flesh and substance to our often made generalizations about addicts' prominent reactions of splitting, projection, impaired reality sense, other primitive defenses and narcissistic rage. She accomplishes this through her compelling observations and descriptions of the very frequent and troublesome transference distortions that occur between patients and staff in methadone clinics. Her clarification that the often observed extreme, intense and labile outbursts by patients in methadone clinics have irrational and overdetermined origins in the patient's past (and are not simply a function of clinic setting or social background), is a helpful reminder to the most seasoned staff member, and may also act as a helpful guide to the novice staff worker in a methadone clinic. Her paper should be required reading for all staff and administrators working in a methadone clinic.

Kaplan presents an in-depth case report about a heroin addict and her family. The detailed clinical description of this woman highlights some of the severe narcissistic disturbances and pathological regression and fixation present in so many addicts. The pathological disturbances of the parents are also well spelled out and give us clear understanding of this patient's developmental failures and troubled identification with her parents. In the absence of mature defenses and an enabling ego (ideal), such patients have few choices but to adopt regressive oral satisfactions.

Finally, Frosch and Milkman in their paper discuss their research findings which appear to support the observations of Wieder and Kaplan, Khantzian and others, that selection of specific "drug of choice" is determined by particular ego vulnerabilities, dispositions and drive strengths.[1] The drugs are used by such individuals syntonically to either augment or bolster certain modes and styles of adaptation, or to compensate for certain ego deficiencies. Frosch and Milkman's findings and their conclusions further lead them to concur with Wieder and Kaplan that the drugs are used to induce ego states reminiscent of a similar state in earlier developmental phases (along lines proposed by Mahler). Whereas the heroin addict uses opiates to achieve a "narcissistic blissful" state of union dating back to a very early phase of development, the amphetamine user takes advantage of the stimulating action of the drug to bolster a grandiose sense of omnipotence through movement and activity akin to the "practicing period" at a slightly later period of development (around one and one-half years old).

DISCUSSION

In the following collection of papers the reader will be rewarded by the richness of insight which a psychodynamic understanding can bring to bear on the drug-problems field. He/she will no doubt also encounter some of the difficulties inherent in an approach which attempts to do justice to human complexity and individuality. As a beginning, one need only note the plethora of terminologies and definitions to conclude, as Dr. Wieder points out in the opening paper, that there is an urgent need to integrate and clarify our definitions and knowledge to date before attempting to open further vistas. Greenspan's paper, for instance, addresses the generic construct of "substance abuse," while Khantzian and Davidson are writing specifically about heroin addicts; Krystal refers to "other drug-dependencies" but appears to center his observations around the problems of alcoholism. This difference in focus leads to the apparently contradictory emphasis on the adaptive advantage of long-acting drugs by Wurmser and Khantzian on the one hand, and of short-acting drugs by Krystal and Raskin on the other. Wieder specifically redefines drug addiction around a concept of compulsiveness in distinction to the traditional criterion of physical dependence; yet Frosch and Milkman in their experimental work based on theoretical conceptualizations similar to Wieder's, define drug dependency operationally in terms of specific amount and frequency of drug use.

---

[1]As indicated in chapter 1, this paper was written before the second meeting which is reported by Woody in chapter 11.

Admittedly, some of these difficulties are only semantic, and other apparent differences stem from preferences in focus. But a close look suggests some basic areas which require fuller consideration before a unitary conceptualization of the problems and issues can be derived. Diagnostic considerations constitute a case in point. Both Wieder and Kaplan consider drug use as symptomatic but not pathognomic, thus underscoring observed diagnostic heterogeneity of drug-using patients, even within a specific type such as narcotic addicts. Wurmser, on the other hand, finds it more useful to consider the varieties of pathological drug use from the base of a common constellation of personality features. Nevertheless, with both formulations, the "drug of choice" phenomenon emerges as a reference point for systematizing observations, and thus provides a common meeting ground. Greenspan's proposition that the specific level of developmental impairment has predictive value in relation to the malignancy of the drug taking, and thus to prognosis, provides another organizing dimension.

The relationship of the drug to the psychopathology of drug users is another aspect of the diagnostic puzzle. Khantzian suggests that drug use and dependency tend to mask the nature of the underlying psychopathology, and that diagnostic assessment must be deferred until drug-taking behavior is under control. Wurmser, on the other hand, tends to view drug use as "coextensive" with the pathology, and as such, part and parcel of the dynamic and structural vicissitudes which constitute the specific nature of compulsive drug use. Frosch and Milkman touch on what seems implied by the foregoing, which is the very difficult problem of distinguishing the effects of drug use from its causes. Their study provides a graphic illustration of the sensitive interactions of drug and ego functions by demonstrating statistically significant changes in ratings on a wide range of intrapsychic functions following doses of drugs which are minuscule by street standards. In different terms, Greenspan makes a similar point in his discussion of the interactive aspects of drug effect and ego organizations.

If the authors have technical differences of formulation or definition, there is nonetheless a welcome unanimity and explicitness in their recommendations for treatment. The shared mandate of all the participants in the technical review and in this monograph is, above all, to provide input which will be applicable toward a remedy for what everyone agrees is a painful and costly human problem. In their statement of the problem, the authors' collective dictum is straightforward: That social and other factors notwithstanding, compulsive drug use and addiction in our society are indicative of psychological disturbance, which in the majority of instances, is profound.

Several of the authors comment on public reluctance to accept this position. Davidson notes that the wish to locate the cure for addictive illness outside the patient's psyche (e.g., with drug therapies alone, or via legal sanctions) indicates the same proclivity which in the patient we identify as denial. Wurmser widens the horizon of social commentary in drawing attention to all forms of externalization, including but not limited to drug use, as the defense of our times. "In a sense," Wurmser writes, "the addict—like the paranoid—has been most successful in making the world serve his inner defense . . . in forcing his surroundings near and far to play their roles in what is originally an internal conflict."

Each of the authors has courageously addressed the problem of what constitutes realizable and adequate treatment. There appears to be a consensus in this monograph that psychoanalytic insights rigorously applied to the problems of addiction can make a major contribution to the treatment of individuals in trouble with drugs. The specific elaborations on treatment issues can be summarized in terms of four constituents: these include, 1) multiple modality approaches to do justice to the complexity and multiplicity of determinants in pathological drug use; 2) a bi-phasic therapeutic strategy consisting first of interim measures for keeping patients available and intact until the second phase of longer range work in psychotherapy can be firmly established; 3) the use of treatment personnel who are fully trained and who hold the particular qualities needed for this kind of work; and 4) specificity of diagnosis and treatment planning.

On hindsight, this prescription may seem self-evident. Yet, although many current treatment options offer one or more of these constituents, rarely do they combine all of them.

The call for multiple approaches in treatment heralds a refreshing eclecticism which need not undermine the integrity of a unitary theoretical framework. For example, Wurmser suggests utilizing combinations of individual, group, and family therapy, together with supportive medication, hospitalization, and vocational and other forms of social counseling. Kaplan's detailed case presentation provides an illustration of the flexible use of a wide variety of resources brought to bear on a whole family. Krystal offers an example of the successful use of a team approach in the treatment of alcoholics, particularly in the interest of utilizing therapeutically the otherwise destructive transference splitting which occurs so often with clinic or institutional patients.

The second constituent of treatment, which overlaps the first, counsels the need for, as Khantzian puts it, "initial treatment interventions to provide the structure and time that make the understanding and management of the addict's problems possible." Such interventions serve to take into account the issue stressed repeatedly in these papers, namely, the inadequacy of internal psychological structures in so many pathological drug users. Such interventions may include any or all of the multiple approaches considered above, and Greenspan adds an additional dimension, in focusing consideration on why such individuals are particularly vulnerable to external environmental influences.

The second phase of the bi-phasic approach is, of course, the crux of the treatment, namely, long-term psychotherapy. The necessity to think in terms of lengthy treatment, including the dependable availability of the primary therapist, is particularly well elaborated by Krystal as he details the specific unfolding of issues in the treatment process. He reminds us of the often misunderstood fact that as old defenses are given up, the patient appears to himself and to the world to be "worse" as he begins to experience his own feelings and impulses which were heretofore undefined, externalized, or otherwise thwarted. And it is particularly for this reason that at this point "dependence upon the therapist is extreme, and no substitutes are acceptable."

Thus the third constituent emerges as the elaboration of those processes which must occur in psychotherapy proper, and in that context also, the qualities the therapist must bring to the task.

Khantzian discusses the delicate balances that the effective therapist must maintain in his work with such patients. There must be confrontation, but it must be done with consistent and empathic respect for the tenuousness of those mechanisms of defense by which self-esteem is maintained, however troublesome or offensive they may appear to the casual observer. Similarly, the therapist must tread the fine line between closeness and distance as problems with primary relationships emerge into the therapeutic relationship. Khantzian's formulation regarding drugs as substituting for defective and absent defenses, and safeguarding against overwhelming and disorganizing affect, lead logically to advocating the use of psychotropic agents as part of the therapy while issues of extremes of self-indulgence and self-denial are negotiated. Kaplan, Krystal and Wurmser all cover similar territory. The modifications of a strictly transference-oriented approach are stressed with the requirement that the therapist play a real role in the patient's life, including limit setting, but again, they caution against the naive application of other extremes. Thus, Wurmser, too, stresses balances, between nurturing and engulfment, between active and intrusive intervention, and between emotional distance and availability. Davidson's contributions are particularly important in this context since they provide detailed consideration of the counter-transference pitfalls in this kind of treatment. Not only is this worth stressing to the seasoned therapist, but it highlights a major pitfall that undertrained staff may be subject to, namely, adroit manipulations whereby staff members come to act out the roles projectively assigned to them by their patients. The fourth constituent in a sense brings the prescription for treatment into full circle. Whatever generalizations have been advanced, the appreciation of the uniqueness of individuals is sustained in stressing the necessity for individualized diagnosis and treatment planning.

Together the present collection of papers is testimony to contemporary theoretical and technical developments which have provided the vehicle for the authors of this monograph to rise to the challenge of comprehending and providing a sober and realistic direction for this difficult and many-sided problem. What has evolved here is not just another would-be panacea but rather the application of a particular perspective, individually developed, toward a common goal. The result at this early juncture appears promising, that a psychodynamic psychology can provide a powerful tool in the further evolution of training, treatment and prevention.

REFERENCES

Chein, I., Gerard, D.L., Lee, R.S., and Rosenfeld, E. *The Road to H.* New York: Basic Books, 1964.

Fenichel, O. *The Psychoanalytic Theory of Neurosis.* New York: W.W. Norton, 1945.

Gerard, D.L., and Kornetsky, C. Adolescent opiate addiction: A case study. *Psychiatr Q*, 28:367-380, 1954.

Glover, E. On the etiology of drug addiction. In: *On the Early Development of Mind.* New York: International Universities Press, 1956.

Hartmann, D. A study of drug taking adolescents. *Psychoanal Study Child*, 24:384-398, 1969.

Hendin, H. Students on heroin. *J Nerv Ment Dis*, 158:240-255, 1974.

Khantzian, E.J. A preliminary dynamic formulation of the psychopharmacologic action of methadone. In: Proc. Fourth National Methadone Conference, San Francisco, January 1972.

————. Opiate addiction: A critique of theory and some implications for treatment. *Am J Psychother*, 28:59-70, 1974.

————. Self selection and progression in drug dependence. *Psychiatry Dig*, 36:19-22, 1975.

Krystal, H., and Raskin, H.A. *Drug Dependence. Aspects of Ego Functions.*
Detroit: Wayne State University Press, 1970.
Milkman, H., and Frosch, W.A. On the preferential abuse of heroin and am-
phetamine. *J Nerv Ment Dis,* 156:242-248, 1973.
Radford, P., Wiseberg, S., and Yorke, C. A study of "main line" heroin addic-
tion. *Psychoanal Study Child,* 27:156-180, 1972.
Rado, S. The psychoanalysis of pharmacothymia. *Psychoanal Q,* 2:1, 1933.
_____ . Narcotic bondage. A general theory of the dependence on narcotic
drugs. *Am J Psychiat,* 114:165, 1957.
Savit, R.A. Extramural psychoanalytic treatment of a case of narcotic addic-
tion. *J Am Psychoanal Assoc,* 2:494, 1954.
Wieder, H., and Kaplan, E. Drug use in adolescents. *Psychoanal Study Child,*
24:399, 1969.
Wurmser, L. Methadone and the craving for narcotics: Observations of patients
on methadone maintenance in psychotherapy. In: Proc. Fourth National
Methadone Conference, San Francisco, January 1972.
_____ . Psychoanalytic considerations of the etiology of compulsive drug
use. *J Amer Psychoanal Assoc,* 22:820-843, 1974.
Yorke, C. A critical review of some psychoanalytic literature on drug addic-
tion. *Brit J Med Psychol,* 43:141, 1970.
Zinberg, N.E. Addiction and ego function. *Psychoanal Study Child,* 30:567-
588, 1975.

CHAPTER 3

Needed: A Theory (An Historical Perspective)

Herbert Wieder, M.D.

Why, in the presence of a vast amount of data obtained from clinical experiences, experimental studies, statistical analyses and research in the basic sciences, has the enigma of drug use not been more rewardingly clarified? A cursory review of my experiences extending back to 1946 suggested their presentation to illuminate an important obstacle to clarification. If some lessons could be learned from the past and delineated, fresh ideas might be released. "Even," as Freud said, "if we cannot see things clearly, we will at least see clearly what the obstacles are." (Freud 1926, p. 124).

HISTORICAL REVIEW

Participating in a conference on the application of psychodynamic theory to the treatment of opiate addiction evoked a feeling of déjà vu. In 1946 a group of clinical staff at the former U.S. Public Health Service Hospital at Lexington, Kentucky, met regularly to discuss the addict patients. Extended over a 3-year period, these meetings were supplemented by consultative discussions with psychoanalysts. Although new to this clinical problem, all staff were eager and energetic.

From the beginning we were confronted by what we came to learn were the vicissitudes of aggression and libido, deviant ego development, disturbed object relationships, superego malformation, and psychodynamic conflicts influenced by intoxicants. With the help of the psychoanalytic literature and consultants, we also rediscovered observations and conclusions of our predecessors.

26

Since we were studying addicts, we thought our findings related to narcotic addicts in particular. We were gradually disabused by the recognition that after detoxification, addicts were people demonstrating the whole gamut of non-addict psychopathology (Kolb and Himmelsbach 1938; Pescor 1939).

However, we did query and speculate on the applicability of our findings to treatment rationale. This led to devising what were considered innovative approaches in those days. Later in the 1960's many of the same proposals were rediscovered by others to reappear on the scene as "new" modalities. For example, external "support of the superego" represented by Kentucky's so called Blue Grass Law was one. Similar to it was New York State's later voluntary incarceration in lieu of conviction; prolonged hospitalization at Lexington as an "ego support for dependency needs" was advised; group and individual psychotherapy were encouraged; a pilot Narcotics Anonymous, a spin-off from Alcoholics Anonymous under the aegis of the Salvation Army, was a forerunner to Synanon; different modes of detoxification were explored; confrontation groups were formed. All of these therapeutic plans derived from the application of implications from psychodynamics to the treatment of drug addicts.

Each approach in time returned minimal gains. The inapplicability of a mass-scale approach, as if addiction were a unitary syndrome, became apparent. The inappropriateness of prescribing treatment for symptoms of indeterminate etiology surfaced. The dismal specter of relapse underscored our ineffectiveness in helping patients achieve and maintain a drug-free life. We could explain neither our therapeutic impotence nor our successes because we weren't clear about what we were treating.

Most everyone knew that only after detoxification did the therapeutic struggle for sober, mental equilibrium begin. Therapy, however, could be no more sophisticated, innovative, or successful for these patients specifically than for the general psychiatric population without drug use symptomatology. In addition, the only special treatment unique to drug addiction was the process of detoxification. This is equally true today.

The absence of experienced and analytically sophisticated psychiatrists, who might have reformulated simplistic and illusory premises, handicapped the therapeutic aspect of Lexington's function. Although psychoanalytic treatment itself was not particularly indicated, rather, a sound psychoanalytic viewpoint was needed to orient the conceptualization of drug use in the spectrum of human behavior and to unify the avalanche of research findings.

Insight into the deeper questions of why drugs existed in a person's life was needed. Toward that end the U.S. Public Health Service would have underwritten analytic training for suitable personnel willing to remain in the Service. That program did not materialize.

Unfortunately, and unjustly, Lexington's therapeutic failures became more of public and medical world knowledge than did important research and observational contributions, which were often unnoticed.

The research department had the advantage of a Governmental mandate to conduct basic and original research into narcotic addiction. In those days "narcotic" was a legal term as much as a pharmacological one. All substances subject to control by the Bureau of Narcotics were loosely called narcotics, and possession or use was considered a narcotic violation. The confusion and equation of legal and pharmacologic terms became fixed in the public's mind. For the first time pharmacology, neurophysiology, neuropharmacology, experimental neurology, biochemistry and—what would nowadays be difficult—human experimentation were brought to bear on the phenomenology of drug use.

Objective evidence, as contrasted to widely divergent clinical opinions, personal attitudes, and mythology, about drugs and users was obtained. Much of the data is still valid and must be integrated, not ignored, into present-day thinking concerning drug use.

From the physiological, pharmacological, and clinical psychiatric investigations a wealth of information was garnered. For example: The abstinence syndrome of opiates was documented and classified; physical dependence and tolerance were demonstrated as consequences of habitual use and not the causes of, or synonyms for, addiction. In the attempt to define "addiction," however, the researchers somewhat arbitrarily decided that the presence of physical dependence was a necessary concomitant for a user to be considered "addicted" to an opiate. The criterion, physical dependence, was incorporated into a general definition of "addiction," "addictive" and "addicted" and led to many of the prevailing difficulties in conceptualizing and defining drugs and their use. It posed the puzzle, for example: Is an addict who has been detoxified still an addict?

This restricted definition of addiction was a concept too narrow to be applied to the broad spectrum of use, drugs, and users that came to light. Isbell was still at work on a definition in 1970. As an internist, he had recognized early what most psychologically minded researchers later came to believe, namely, that addiction was best conceived as a kind of compulsion to alter a state of mind, not a physical state exemplified by physical dependence (Isbell and

Chrusciel 1970). The observation that drugs are not indiscriminately chosen or freely interchangeable contradicted a commonly held belief. Left to freedom of choice, users establish a "drug of choice," or preference. Together with Kaplan in 1969, I reported on this phenomenon. Drug free did not mean cured or healthy; physical dependence especially in the younger age groups did not necessarily augur the severe psychopathology characteristic of the older, chronic user (Wieder and Kaplan 1969). These emerging distinctions were ill-served by a definition of addiction restricted to physical dependence.

Marihuana users did not fit the concept of addiction which stressed physiological concomitants along with a compulsion (Kolb 1938). Marihuana habitues were different from morphinists, and most of the former did not even use opiates occasionally (Pescor 1943). The U.S. Public Health Service argued for decrimininalization of marihuana in 1947 because neither the users nor the substance conformed to the working definition of addict or addiction; nor for that matter did cocaine, mescaline, and other substances. The close causal connection that was believed to exist between crime and use of drugs was disproved along with the myth of marihuana as the steppingstone to heroin. However, even when these points were aired by the "President's Commission on Crime," they were not widely accepted. The disavowal of myth-puncturing data was, and still is, evident. Questions remained. How was use of marihuana and other substances to fit into the concept of drug addiction? Where did alcohol and alcoholism fit?

Very few opiate addicts voluntarily coming off the street demonstrated strong signs of an objective abstinence syndrome (Kolb and Himmelsbach 1938). On the other hand, many who used barbiturates to supplement their drug need developed severe, sometimes fatal reactions to their hospitalization, before the barbiturate abstinence syndrome was recognized.

Further Lexington contributions established how to detoxify, and the need to confirm the presence of physical dependency before detoxification. Methadone research and clinical trials on our withdrawal service developed methadone's status as an agent superior to morphine for detoxification from opiates. The research division also predicted the chaos that has now occurred if methadone were not considered as equivalent to morphine in its effects and consequences (Isbell et al. 1947).

The amount of data did not receive the wide acceptance they deserved. Lexington was producing objective evidence and was being ignored or repudiated by clinical impressionists. I reported on two contradictions to clinical impressions. Demerol was proclaimed in clinical medicine as non-addicting, except to people who had abused morphine. Even after reporting (Wieder 1946) addiction of the first few primary Demerol users the myth of its non-addicting quality remained. A second report (Wieder 1949) repudiated insulin as a safe, good treatment for the abstinence syndrome, an example of a treatment elaboration based on unconfirmed clinical impressions. (Insulin therapy of schizophrenia had been developed by Sakel [1930] on the basis of the good results he thought he had observed in the treatment of the abstinence syndrome.) A later, more current example in my judgment is the misuse of methadone for maintenance, based on illusory premises and ignoring the implication of its interchangeability with opiates (Dole and Nyswander 1965).

The need for rigorous controls in the study of drug use and users was ignored by many. As one small example, many people believed they could detoxify a physically dependent user on an open ward. All of the observational safeguards necessary to demonstrate physical dependence (Kolb and Himmelsbach 1938) during the first 36 hours of hospitalization were ignored. Therefore the efficacy of a detoxification procedure could not even be demonstrated as needed. No therapeutic program for drug-using patients can be assessed without strict safeguards.

But with all its data, Lexington could not formulate psychologically true definitions or a theory of addiction that could apply to the total scene of man's involvement with drugs. Lexington's imprint on the thinking about the problem remained consistent with a medical model of illness.

Apart from its paucity and deficiencies in the type of data Lexington was developing, the psychoanalytic and psychiatric literature prior to 1960 was limited in scope by the (N.B. upper class) socioeconomic type and small number of patients treated and reported (see Bibliography). Drug addiction was predominantly viewed as an impulse disorder and implicitly referred to opiates. Though the analytic reports were informative, the formulations and psychodynamics described could have been applied to many who were not addicts. Importantly, however, many who reported cases would draw attention to phenomenology of non-drug-using patients who behaved toward objects, food, love, fetishes, and tobacco, for example, "like drug addicts." Freud had once said that masturbation was the first addiction, and all others were substitutes for it (Freud 1897). This may be partially true, but the total dynamics are more complex.

Although the symptom of drug taking, ranging from benign to

malignant, occurs in patients belonging to all categories of psychiatric classification, analysts maintained a unitary view of drug addiction as a special syndrome. "Addiction" or "addict" meant morphinist; morphinist meant addict, and therefore refractory to analysis. Very few people understood that of all the forms of drug use, use of opiates was the least prevalent, though perhaps the most dramatic and publicized. No encompassing theory of addiction or drug use was developed by the analysts, even though Rado's paper of 1933, addressed to the fundamental questions of what is an addict and why do people use drugs, was a promising start (Rado 1933). While Lexington staff suffered from an absence of psychoanalytic perspectives, the psychoanalysts suffered from an absence of comprehensive, objective clinical data.

Rado's insight that "not the toxic agent but the impulse to use it is what makes an addict of a given person" (1933. p.2) attempted to redress the distortion of viewpoint that the drug "took" the person. Freud, before Rado, had expressed the notion that some peculiarity in the user accounts for addiction. The insights lay dormant until rediscovered in the 1950's and 1960's when social alarm refocused analytic thinking onto drug users (Savitt 1963). Rado's insight could have been the cornerstone for a theory in the 1930's. It is the necessary starting point. I believe any theory that ignores that insight and its implications will be inadequate and will permit the perpetuation of confusion in conceptualization.

In the 1950's drug use seemed to erupt on an international scale, forcing clinical attention upon psychiatrists and psychoanalysts with little but their own limited experience and education in the drug scene. The model of adult opiate addicts and their refractoriness to psychoanalytic treatment dominated professional thinking, and few people wanted to treat drug-using patients. At the same time sociologists, educators, psychologists, penologists, clergymen, and opportunists exploded on the scene with their own brands of cure and salvation. Though much of this furor could be seen as the anxious cries of a threatened and uninformed society, confusion was rampant among the professionals. At that time psychoanalysis and psychiatry had lost whatever prestige they had in this area by default. Because of the disappointment of unrealistic therapeutic expectations the public harbored and the realistic ignorance which they professed, by their disinterest in treating drug-using patients psychiatrists and analysts were viewed as just another source of unhelpful opinion.

I refer you to the "Conferences on Drug Addiction Among Adolescents" (1953) held at the New York Academy of Medicine in 1951 and 1952. These conferences were called to meet the emergency of "drug addicts loose in New York City"—an alarm that had been sounded in a 1921 conference and again in the 1960's. Wild estimates ranging from 2,000 to 250,000 appear often and with the flimsiest basis of demonstrable evidence. A host of talented and experienced people from various disciplines—sociology, penology, psychiatry, public health—met and presented their data in familiar sounding terminology. However, each discipline had its own set of meanings and definitions. Those who represented the legal professions viewed addiction as a criminal act; for them a drug was a drug only if the substance was prohibited by the law. For sociologists, addiction was an illness produced by availability of substances in the context of socioeconomic factors. Psychiatrists described addiction as the consequence of an impulse disorder. Everyone's aim was to "cure," meaning to "stamp out drugs." No collaborative effort was possible, each discipline vying for dominance, and no psychological base to unify the findings could be proposed.

WHAT IS NEEDED

The same lack of definition persists in the present. Everyone has his own idea about the problem and will continue to perpetuate confusion unless areas of agreement are found for formulations.

A working theory should encompass what has been clinically and experimentally confirmed, explain a good deal, and have some predictive reliability. Such a theory would have precluded, among other things, excessive governmental expenditures on poorly conceived programs whose failures were predictable. Theory would also facilitate better diagnostic discrimination for the rational prescription of available treatment modalities.

A Panel (1975) at the American Psychoanalytic Association disseminated drug-related clinical experiences and observations in research projects. Levels of experience and sophistication were widely disparate, and the infrequency of meetings prevented developing a cohesive accumulation of theory and experience.

Results of a study group of the Association for Child Analysis were reported by Dora Hartmann (1969). A group of child analysts studying drug-using adolescents experienced difficulties at the onset by a confusion of terminology and orientation. A profitable year studying cases ended up rediscovering much that was already known. Modifications of therapeutic technique, however, were determined by the dynamic and diagnostic considerations of each case. Reasonable successes were achieved with some.

Rediscovery is certainly at times valuable; for many it is educational or confirmatory of past data. But it can also become an endless repetition. It is my belief that we are less in need of data than of a systematic examination of what is available.

From the mass of data extant, some formulations based on psychoanalytic concepts could and should be tentatively structured, initiating a common language. The problem of definition, terminology, conceptualization, and theory formation is central to our inability to penetrate the enigma. As things stand now, everyone has his own theory, and that is as good as none. All statistics, proposals, claims and counterclaims should be reviewed from a base of unified, realistic definition.

Kaplan and I (1969, 1971) have offered such a tentative set of formulations, derived from a study in depth of the drug of choice phenomenon, which are explanatory and predictive. Definitions of "drug" and "use" and terminology for classification of users are consistent with psychoanalytic concepts. Our theory and formulations are in accord with psychoanalytic hypotheses, the clinical scene, and the overall human behavior with drugs. Formulations applicable to all phases of life place drug use into the spectrum of human behavior from so-called normal to pathological. We claim no preemption of a theory with our contribution. However, it may be viewed as a working model of what a group of analysts could collaboratively derive.

The aim of finding practical application of theory to the treatment of opiate addiction raises a number of questions. Does it imply that dynamic theory is not currently applied to treatment? Surely not, since any regimen that could be dignified with the term "rational therapy" would be devised or prescribed on inferences from a patient's psychodynamics and diagnosis. Certainly the analytic literature is replete with examples of modification of therapeutic technique as a function of a patient's developmental deviations and needs (Maenchen 1970; Eissler 1958). Any inferences from psychodynamics as applied to treatment, however, are specific for an individual patient, not generalized for presenting symptomatology per se.

Is narcotic addiction again being singled out as a unitary syndrome, as distinct from symptomatic behavior of diverse etiology? Is there an implication that psychoanalytic theory would illuminate homogeneous psychodynamics differentiating opiate addicts from other chronic drug-using patients? Although a patient's preferential use of opium can reveal something about his manner of conflict solution, we are not informed by that preference of the urgency with which he seeks it. The use of terms such as "narcotic addiction" and "addict" suggest the persistent presence of a sterotype image that ignores the spectrum of use and user. If we think therefore that by applying our knowledge of psychodynamics to the problem of narcotic addiction we improve our therapeutic capabilities, we have a skewed view. It is inconceivable that a single-minded emphasis in any relevant discipline will unravel the puzzle. Psychoanalysis, however, offers the most comprehensive view of human behavior and development, the most fruitful frame of reference or underlying orientation to tie data from many disciplines together. As both a contributing collaborator with his own data, and an organizer and synthesizer of diverse data, the psychoanalyst with his unique viewpoint will contribute most in the area of formulation and theory development.

Before innovative procedures are proposed or programed, serious attention should first focus on formulating the problem, rigorously adhering to psychoanalytic concepts. I would propose a multidisciplined "Think Tank," chaired by a psychoanalyst, to sift, evaluate, and structure different levels of information. With the millions of dollars wasted on many wild projects in the past, the cost of such sober reflection would be the least expensive for potentially rich results, and the most innovative approach in the long run.

When our national crusade on cancer was launched, the British Government wisely heeded the advice of its chief scientific adviser and refused to join. His opinion about cancer is equally applicable to any crusade mounted against the drug crisis: "In my view, any campaign which sets out to buy a cure for cancer without the most careful and thorough preliminary long term planning is in danger of encouraging mediocrity and the routine pursuit of ideas which may long since have ceased to be fertile" (Zuckerman 1972).

REFERENCES

Conferences on Drug Addiction Among Adolescents. New York: Blakiston Division, McGraw Hill, 1953.

Dole, V.P., and Nyswander, M. A Medical Treatment for Diacetyl morphine (Heroin) Addiction. A Clinical Trial with Methadone Hydrochloride. *JAMA*, 193:646-650, 1965.

Eissler, K. Notes on Problems of Technique in the Psychoanalytic Treatment of Adolescents: with Some Remarks on Perversions. *Psychoanal Study Child*, 13:223-254, 1958.

Freud, S. *The Origins of Psycho-analysis. Letters to Wilhelm Fliess*, #79. Marie Bonaparte, Anna Freud, Ernst Kris, eds. New York: Basic Books, 1953.

Freud, S. *Inhibition, Symptoms, and Anxiety.* SE XX. London: Hogarth Press, 1926, p. 124.

Hartmann, D. A Study of Drug Taking Adolescents. *Psychoanal Study Child*, 24:384-398, 1969.

Isbell, H. et al. Tolerance and Addiction Liability of 6-Dimethylamino-4-4-Diphenyl-Heptanone-3 (Methadone). *JAMA*, 135:888-894, 1947.

Isbell, H., and Chrusciel, T.L. Dependence Liability of Non-Narcotic Drugs. Supplement #43 to *Bulletin of WHO*, Geneva, 1970.

Kaplan, E.H., and Wieder, H. *Drugs Don't Take People—People Take Drugs.* Secaucus, N.J.: Lyle Stuart, 1974.

Kolb, L. Marijuana. *Federal Probation*, July 1938.

Kolb, L., and Himmelsbach, C.K. Clinical Studies in Drug Addiction. *Am J Psychiatry*, 94:4, 1938.

Kolb, L., and Himmelsbach, C.K. Clinical Studies of Drug Addiction. Supplement #128, *Public Health Service Reports*, 1938.

Maenchen, A. On the Technique of Child Analysis in Relation to Stages of Development. *Psychoanal Study Child*, 25:175-200, 1970.

Pescor, M.J. The Kolb Classification of Drug Addicts. Supplement #155, *Public Health Service Reports*, 1939.

Pescor, M.J. A Statistical Analysis of the Clinical Records of Hospitalized Drug Addicts. Supplement #143, *Public Health Service Reports*, 1943.

Rado, S. The Psychoanalysis of Pharmacothymia (Drug Addiction) 1. The Clinical Picture. *Psychoanal Q*, Vol II, No. 1:1-23, 1933.

Sakel, M. Theorie der Sucht. *Zeitschrift für den gesamelten Neurologische u. Psychologische*, 129:639, 1930.

Savitt, R.A. Psychoanalytic Studies on Addiction, Ego Structure in Narcotic Addiction. *Psychoanal Q*, 32:43-57, 1963.

Wieder, H. Addiction to Meperidine Hydrochloride (Demerol Hydrochloride). *JAMA*, 132:1066-1068, 1946.

Wieder, H. Objective Evaluation of Insulin Therapy of the Morphine Abstinence Syndrome. *J Nerv Ment Dis*, Vol. 110, 1:26-35, 1949.

Wieder, H., and Kaplan, E.H. Drug Use in Adolescents. Psychodynamic Meaning and Pharmacogenic Effect. *Psychoanal Study Child*, 24:399-431, 1969.

Zuckerman, Lord Solly. Cancer Research. *Science*, 178:1184, 1972.

CHAPTER 4

Mr. Pecksniff's Horse?
(Psychodynamics in Compulsive
Drug Use)

Leon Wurmser, M.D.

I would like to thank the research staff at the National Institute
on Drug Abuse for opening a potentially fruitful and important dia-
logue with members of the psychoanalytic community who have
worked intensively and extensively with compulsive drug users.

Since this topic also forms the core of a book I have just completed, I decided I would do most justice by selecting a few pertinent excerpts from that work for presentation here. For brevity, I
leave out supporting evidence and most of the broad theoretical
implications. All of that will be published in, I hope, quite exhaust-
ive form. [1]

Here, the major and encompassing ideas underlying the investigation will be summarized; a brief description of some psychodynamic findings will follow, leading to several recommendations.
Since even this adumbrated presentation is somewhat lengthy, the
following title outline may help the reader:

THE SHIFT IN FOCUS
ANALYSIS OF THE DIRECT ANTECEDENTS
 The Vicious Circle
 Affect Regression and Breakdown of Affect Defense
 The Search for an Affect Defense
 Splitting
 Externalization—The Neglected Defense
 Summary of the Direct Antecedents
SOME COMMENTS ABOUT PREDISPOSITION
TREATMENT
 Psychotherapy
 Large-scale Treatment Policy

---

[1]

THE SHIFT IN FOCUS

The starting point of my reevaluation of some of the common preconceptions about compulsive drug users in general and narcotic addicts in particular was the following distressing experience, repeated many times over the last 12 years since I started working intensively and systematically with all types of what is too loosely called "drug abuse."

At first I was provoked by the habits and attitudes of these patients, feeling that I was dealing indeed with the scum of mankind, feeling anger about being lied to and manipulated, feeling scorn for their flaunting of being "high" and their flouting of all efforts to help them and of all rules we live by.

Yet the more I got to know them, anger, disdain, frustration vanished, and a deep sense of despair and pity broke through. I could hardly find better words than what Faust said entering the dungeons where Margarete was awaiting the dawn and her execution, his almost untranslatable: "The whole depth of human misery grips me" ("Der Menschheit ganzer Jammer fasst mich an"). Often I felt a sense of helplessness, a wish to help, and an ignorance of how to help. The problems of drugs, drug effects, drug prohibition receded, paled compared with the overwhelming problems posed by these patients who sought help, were forced to be treated, fled from help, died.

When I followed the literature, the discussions at scientific conventions, the opinions expressed by friends, in audiences, by lawyers, no suggestions, no help were offered. A vast *terra incognita* was lying before me, covered by such expressions as: "They are just sociopaths!" or "They are not motivated," "the living dead," "the dope fiends." Thus the problem posed itself with glaring sharpness: How can drug abuse be understood from the context of the individual's life experience, from his wishes and fears, from his deficiencies and efficiencies, from his conflicts in past and present—in short, from a psychological point of view. How can these deeper problems be treated?

Thus on the one side we have a relative plethora of pharmacological studies and sociological inquiries, although I do not imply these are redundant, and much more work in these fields should be done. Moreover, the politics and the legal aspects of illegal drug use fill the columns of our newspapers and tax the exegetical skills of self-styled experts of all kinds: lawyers, politicians, policemen and administrators. Many deal seriously and compassionately with the problems, many others make cheap hay from them, but most skim just the surface.

On the other side, drug abuse has remained off the beaten track, where many psychiatric and psychological explorers will not tread. There are good reasons for this: one is precisely the complexity of the problem, namely that psychological factors are so tightly interwoven with sociological, economic, political, and legal factors. Where the values of power, expediency, public success, and cost efficiency are uppermost, the required strategies of manipulation and control become so intermingled with therapeutic considerations that the value of insight, inner change and control, and the methods of introspection and empathy, have perforce to take a back seat. Yet, in all these years that I have consistently devoted a large part of my professional work to these patients I have been struck by this overriding impression: that severe psychopathology was a preexisting condition in those people for whom "drug abuse" became a real problem; that these inner problems were indeed of crucial explanatory importance.

At the same time I noticed resistance against this view, resistance of different content, from different walks of life, of various intensity and origin. Medical colleagues frowned upon it. Psychiatrists doubted it. Even some psychoanalytic friends felt I exaggerated the role of intrapsychic and family problems as compared with social, cultural and political influences. My co-workers in the drug abuse programs were often quite negative about recognizing the psychological problems and—sometimes with some derision—emphasized instead the value of manipulation and exhortation in the form of counseling, the value of external change. The patients themselves very often—though by no means always—put their problems on friends, "bad environment," "curiosity" and "society." Their families regularly did, nearly without fail.

A large role in this negation is played by an antipsychiatric bias on many levels, a prejudice against looking at one's inner life (problems or potentialities), at times so strong that we might call it "psychophobia"—a deep-seated fear of taking emotional factors seriously, *a denial of the importance of emotional conflict*, which haunts drug abusers as well as those dealing with it.

Thus, I decided to collect as much evidence for the importance of psychopathology as I could muster and put it in a reasonable perspective. Obviously many other factors—social, cultural, etc.—are involved, cannot be neglected, have to be weighed, put in relation to the rather crushing weight of personal clinical experience.

This leads to a rather radical refocusing which has only a few precedents, mainly, the work of Krystal and Raskin, Wieder and Kaplan, Khantzian, Frosch.

These reformulations can be summarized in the following five points:

(1) The focus of inquiry and intervention is shifted *from drugs to personality*, from drug use as a social phenomenon which might be relatively easily manipulated, deterred, cured by external means (such as threats, counseling, laws and jails), to drug use as a symptom of a psychological depth dimension which has been up to now only rarely investigated or treated. This implies that psychoanalysis and psychotherapy have to contribute a vastly neglected component to the study and treatment of this mass phenomenon.

At a time when both psychoanalysis and psychiatry are under fire for being irrelevant, moribund or dead, this study is grounded in the *psychoanalytic process of inquiry* in regard to both observation and abstraction. Hence it is no part of the current stampede to get "nothing but Facts . . . imperial gallons of facts," the flight from theoretical constructions and hierarchies of abstractions. Nor does it take any theory as dogma, as more than a form of symbolic representation. Symbols are not facts, but ways to order them— indispensable, but on a different plane of understanding.

(2) Yet this reorientation does not lead to a one-way street. Rather, psychoanalysis as *theory* may in turn benefit from new observations gained in this field. Therefore, the investigation underlying this brief essay, by examining in depth a number of individual cases, tries to deepen, to question and to enlarge some common (and a few less common) psychoanalytic and psychiatric concepts. For example, the phenomena and theories of narcissism and aggression are reevaluated in the light of these experiences. The defense "mechanisms" of denial and externalization and the problems of splitting are examined. Such investigation may lead to a deeper understanding of the quite complex nature of "simple" defense mechanisms and eventually to a hierarchical ordering of them. At the same time these defense mechanisms have to be viewed as patterns of drive gratification, as cognitive forms and basic elements of symbolization, and as fundamental action patterns. [In addition to new thoughts about forms of defense, the book at large, though not this excerpt, attempts, perhaps most importantly, to reexamine the concept of *boundaries and limits*, a notion which proves to be crucial for an understanding of these patients, and attempts to integrate the concept more solidly with current psychoanalytic theory.] Throughout, the affects of guilt and shame, and their archaic precursors, have proven to be of special help for deeper understanding.

(3) By merely differentiating non-intensive from heavy drug use, the sociolegal definition of drug abuse is woefully inadequate for a

psychotherapeutic approach. Instead, the concept of compulsiveness is chosen as operationally most meaningful, both for this particular field and for psychopathology in general. It serves as *the* criterion for "emotionally sick," as proposed by Kubie, not primarily to adjudge whole persons, but single mental acts. To select this specific "elementary particle" as criterion, with its practical, theoretical and axiological implications, appears especially useful and fulfils the crucial criteria for scientific knowledge as set down by Cassirer (1958).

Moreover, compulsiveness emerges as a *relative* property of mental processes: acts (thoughts, feelings, actions etc., and their sequences and patterns) may be *more or less* compulsive, varying from person to person, and within an individual from time to time; acts felt to be absolutely compulsive or absolutely free either do not occur at all or are very rare. Since it is to a large extent observable, this criterion may prove to be particularly helpful for research.

(4) Since drug abuse always involves pharmacological and social factors, it is strategically placed on the crossroads of psychoanalysis and pharmacology, of somatic medicine and general psychiatry. Indeed, the long shadow of drug abuse in human history lies across the crossroads of sociology and politics, of history and philosophy, even of literature and anthropology.

No look at the "hidden dimension" of drug abuse psychodynamics can fail to notice the connections between leading underlying problems in the individual (and this holds true not merely for the drug use itself) and sociocultural and philosophical antitheses, conflicts, contradictions. In a more comprehensive study than presented here much thought will therefore have to be devoted to tracing such lines from the individual to the surrounding circles of etiology, no matter how unspecific such connections remain.

Of particular importance among these connecting threads is the one between various aspects of the superego and axiology. The pathology of ideal formation in compulsive drug abusers reflects a deeper, more general "betrayal of philosophy." Again, there may be mutual illumination between the psychoanalysis of the superego and value philosophical conflicts and hierarchies.

More concretely this leads inevitably into considerations of ethics and legal philosophy. The experiences garnered in psychoanalytic and psychotherapeutic work cast new light on many central questions of these two philosophical fields and hence on the practice of legislation and law enforcement as well.

The psychoanalyst is in a delicate position: she/he cannot advocate specific ethical values; but has to remain, even in clinical work, primarily a scientist who is beholden to one leading value system, viz. that inherent in every scientific method. Yet, as this system applies to psychoanalytic values (integration, freedom of compulsions, integrity and honesty etc.), it has ineluctable effects upon specific decisions of an ethical nature. His central value system is beyond ethics in a narrow sense, but not beyond value philosophy. It also has a most profound influence on ethics, probably as no other area of scientific inquiry.

(5) From all this it becomes obvious that there are, on no level, any simple, quick, easy solutions. The answers to many of the questions lie at this time still out of reach. Glib "either-or" reactions inevitably founder on this *complexity*.

An implication of this complexity is that in no case of severe drug use will one form of treatment suffice. It is typical (quite similar to severe chronic physical illnesses, like leukemia or tuberculosis) that one method of therapy is not enough, that *four to seven (or more) "modalities"* may have to be employed, *concomitantly or sequentially*. It is not at all rare that a therapeutic advance becomes possible only when individual- , group- and family-therapy are combined and often supported by medication or hospitalization, and vocational (and other forms of social) counseling.

The "one-track mentality" is very common and often a cardinal error in the treatment of these patients. Still, even a modality orientation does not do justice to the complexity and quite often may prove disastrous. Not only may it impede the tackling of a patient's severe inner problems, but it may exacerbate a severe "pathology" of treatment programs and systems themselves. In the administration of such programs one often witnesses an "insolence of office," a kind of pathology from people expected to treat it. Further, from insufficient command of complexity, treatment is often "penny wise and pound foolish." By saving in the short run, expenditures grow in the long run massively and outrageously, manifested, for example, in enormous costs of crimes committed by compulsive drug users and due, I believe, mostly to irrational approaches to their problems.

Even individual psychotherapy needs new methods, new parameters, to cope with the peculiar problems of this important group of patients. Conventional psychoanalysis quickly runs into insurmountable difficulties. At the same time some of the basic conditions of psychoanalysis (analysis of transference, countertransference, resistance) remain indispensable.

Recommendations made on the basis of recognizing this hidden, often negated or circumvented issue of compulsive drug use may strike many as revolutionary or puzzling—by those who have not struggled themselves with these patients' problems for many years, who have not been burned many times trying to build up programs for them, and who have not been called to help by the families of these patients in despair. Yet I consider this type of effort very important. A considerable proportion of the population in our culture is involved in mild or severe forms of drug abuse: it may be one-fourth to more than half of the population. Of these, a very large proportion is undoubtedly involved in compulsive forms of drug use (at least between 5 and 10 percent of the population in Western countries) if we include, as we must, alcohol. Therefore, systematic in-depth studies should be considered with the seriousness a social and health problem of such magnitude demands, a problem probably affecting far more people than schizophrenia or most forms of somatic illness.

In addition, the social consequences of this symptom are enormous—another dimension, dealt with by a legal system as ill-suited to deal with the problem as with plague, cholera or depressions.

I hear a loud protest, "You use a medical model; how inappropriate!" My answer is, "Yes, it is primarily a problem of illness and medicine, and more specifically of psychopathology and therefore of psychiatry and psychoanalysis. Logically and historically this makes more sense than any other current claim. It is the only approach which is both humane, seeing and treating this illness like all others, as part of the human condition, and still takes it very seriously—not merely as a social and legal deviance nor as a part of politics and economics, dehumanized to some statistics, nor as a part of physiology, magically overcome by some enzyme repairs and powerful potions." We ought to condemn less and try to understand more.

ANALYSIS OF THE DIRECT ANTECEDENTS

The Vicious Circle

Before the beginning of compulsive drug use, there are clear signs of a serious emotional disorder, one which may be called "the addictive illness" or the signs for an addictive career. We are confronted with the very difficult question how to analyze this complex of phenomena leading to the overt outbreak of the illness. This outbreak especially takes the form of compulsive drug use, but is not always restricted to this symptom. A few equivalents to drug dependency which precede or replace this symptom can be observed repeatedly (violence, other forms of criminality, depression, anxiety attacks, eating disturbances).

The following distinctions emerge: a) A *horizontal plane* ("what goes on in the here and now when I start taking drugs for inner needs") should be distinguished from what we glean from the *vertical plane*, which includes the history, the depth dimension, the predisposition. b) Even on this horizontal level, however, we clearly can distinguish that there are *covert events* which gradually emerge in detailed probing beneath the overt phenomena; these covert processes are partly *preconscious* and relatively easily retrievable, partly *unconscious* and, due to the particular difficulties of psychotherapy or psychoanalysis with these patients, almost inaccessible. c) The conscious and preconscious processes can, without undue problems, be arranged in a fairly regular sequence, a vicious circle, which will be presently outlined. This vicious circle has, as all psychopathology to some extent, a particularly strong self-perpetuating quality, a feeding on itself. d) When we explore the underlying dynamics of the single elements of such a cycle, we discover that all of them are themselves already *compromise formations*, partial conflict solutions. The entire vicious circle thus presents itself as a *complex series of compromise solutions.* e) Next we need to recognize and define distinctly the underlying constituent components: What exactly are the unconscious impulses, wishes, drive components? What exactly are the defenses? How do the defenses themselves reflect instinctual processes? And: What are structural defects —neither defense nor instinctual drive? f) In answering some of these questions we get onto very slippery terrain and are in danger of sliding into pseudoexplanatory concepts. We come face to face with something which Roy Schafer (1968) rightly complained about: ". . . many of the familiar descriptive and explanatory terms of psychoanalysis are global terms, and, if used without further specification and qualification, they limit or distort perception and conceptualization of the phenomena" (p. 100). The notions of narcissism, denial, splitting, aggression proved to become names that were called by Szasz (1957) "panchresta," catch-all terms, too broad, playing into the need for complaisance and a sense of knowledge, but becoming imprecise, even contradictory cliches. At the same time they could not be discarded by any means. They are, as the term "panchreston" connotes, overly general, they need further specifications, redefinitions, and occasionally new contents. At times the attempts to do this are provisional first trials at differentiating what seems well covered with the broad notions.

But to start we have to examine the more overt, less arcane vicious circle which is accessible to any careful ("microscopic") inspection. To illustrate, I use the near verbatim account by a patient of how he experienced his going to the Bowery at age 19

and getting drunk, and how this was identical with many events
with alcohol before, with drugs later on, a sequence which I could
witness as well right in the sessions.

(1) It starts out with "any big event whether I succeed or I fail;
it has the same aftermath: sadness, letdown, loneliness." In all
patients it is some form of disappointment—realistic or in fantasy,
a letdown from an expectation which may be justified or, more
often, vastly exaggerated, an expectation usually of one's own
grandeur, far less commonly a disappointment about someone else.
This sudden plummeting of self-esteem is best called a *narcissistic
crisis*.

(2) The next step is that the feelings become overwhelming,
global, archaic, physically felt, cannot be articulated in words. "I
feel a foreign power in me which I cannot name; all barriers are
gone." The patients describe an uncontrollable, intense sense of
rage or shame or despair, etc. This is clearly an *affect regression*
and brings a generalization and totalization of these very archaic,
often preverbal affects (cf. especially Krystal). It is a *breakdown of
affect defense*.

(3) What happens next is least clear. The affect disappears; only a
vague, but unbearable tension remains; there may be a longing, a
frantic search for excitement and relief, a sense of aimless, intolerable restlessness, a craving (not unlike the one later seen in acute
withdrawal). Instead of the prior feeling we hear: "I thought about
myself as something else, as an object, as a character in a book, that
I was creating the story about myself, a novel. I am not even
actually aware of the pain anymore; it is not you, it is a character in
a book you are creating. My whole life is so: a part who acts and a
part who observes." The intellectual, observing part is not really
alive, the acting one lives. Like Alexander the Great comparing
Achilles with Homer, our patient states: "It is better to *be* the
character than to *write* about him in a novel"—better to act than to
observe. It is important for us to notice the *split*, reminiscent of the
one observed in severe states of depersonalization. This splitting
recurs in many forms in our patients. In the passage just quoted it is
between observing (and controlling) versus acting in a particular
way, which we shall study shortly. More typically it is between the
most troublesome feelings held down, suppressed, disregarded, the
inner problems in general, and a facade, an illusion of being all
right. Or: the problem lies in the body, outside. I believe the split
necessitates above all a *massive denial* of inner reality, specifically
of the overwhelming affects. Other defenses—e.g., negation, avoidance, repression and projection—seem to operate as well, but they
pale beside the role of denial in the exact sense: "Disavowal or

denial as originally described by Freud involves, not an absence or distortion of actual perception, but rather a failure to fully appreciate the significance or implications of what is perceived"—especially of affects (Trunnell and Holt 1974). What is important for us is the phenomenological evidence of many forms of massive splits, accompanied by unconscious denial, by an "invalidating fantasy," and by a partial acknowledgment.

(4) There is a wild drivenness for *action*, for seeking an external *concrete* solution to the internal (and denied) conflict. "It was unbearable; I had to do something external to change the situation—no matter what." Violence, arrest, drugs—the specific *modus* of this *defense by externalization* is actually not even terribly relevant at a given moment for the patient: *the defense by concrete action on the outside which magically changes life* is what counts.

(5) "It was something fascinating when I went to the Bowery. The position was appealing: to destroy myself, to be a bum. It was sheer *self-destructiveness.*" In other moments it was murderous anger. Again, as Anna Freud and many others observed: aggression, especially directed against the self, becomes an inevitable link in the chain. Our paradigmatic case also notes: "I progress, and suddenly I have the urge to break out, to destroy everything I have built up, and then I am completely down for a month and slowly build it (self-esteem, social accomplishment) up again."

This fifth step is the involvement of *aggression*, usually by "breaking out," transgressing boundaries, violating social limits, attacking others, destroying oneself, hurting and being hurt, humiliating others and being shamed.

(6) "When despair takes over, the question of honesty becomes ridiculous." The drowning man has commonly little regard for questions of ethics, of integrity. Conscience becomes utterly irrelevant. Trustworthiness, reliability, commitments to others are acknowledged, and yet made meaningless, treated as if of absolutely no importance whatsoever. Again I believe there is a *profound splitting of the superego*, usually accompanied above all by denial, but also by projection and externalization.

No compulsive drug use (except perhaps for one commonly not recognized as such, like compulsive smoking) goes without this superego split.

(7) "When I have broken out, there is so much enjoyment and excitement, that everything appears okay. I am satisfied then: I feel sheltered. I am acknowledged: the world owes me a living. I get something for nothing, and I deserve it." It is pleasure of many forms—*entitlement* above all—which forms the end point of the cycle.

Let us summarize what we have found so far: It is a series of conflicts, actuated in an acute crisis, which forms *the* specific cause. This specific cause is the following circular constellation: It starts out 1) with the *narcissistic crisis*, leading 2) to overwhelming affects, to an *affect regression*, a totalization and radicalization of these feelings. 3) As directed affect defenses the closely related phenomena of *splitting* ("ego splits") and fragmentation are deployed: the defense, mainly in the form of *denial*, but also of repression and other "mechanisms," is carried out partly by psychological means alone, partly and secondarily by pharmacological propping up (pharmacogenic defense). 4) Denial requires an additional form of defense, the element most specific in this series of seven, defense by *externalization*, the importance of reasserting magical (narcissistic) power by external action—including taking magical "things" such as drugs. 5) This reassertion of power by externalization requires the use of archaic forms of *aggression*, of outwardly attacking and self-destructive forms of sado-masochism. 6) In most cases this is only possible by a sudden *splitting of the superego* and other defenses against superego functions. 7) The final point is the enormous *pleasure* and gratification which this complex of compromise solutions of various instinctual drives with various defenses brings about. Most importantly the acute narcissistic conflict appears resolved—for the moment. But, as Rado described, the patient is caught in a vicious circle: "The elation had augmented the ego [now we would say the self] to gigantic dimensions and had almost eliminated reality; now just the reverse state appears, sharpened by the contrast. The ego is shrunken, and reality appears exaggerated in its dimensions" (1933). The patient is not merely back where he started, but on a yet much lower level of self-esteem.

What I have called "the vicious circle" is represented in the following model.

It is important to consider the probability that *each of the seven* components of the circle is already in itself a *compromise formation, a derivative of impulse, defense and defect (or deficiency).*

We have to keep this in mind and try to analyze this unconscious substratum as well. That part is most difficult and uncertain in its outcome.

Here still another objection will be raised: What is so distinctive about this League of Seven to make them the culprits in the problem posed? Do we not all undergo narcissistic crises, and are severe narcissistic disorders not even the daily bread of all psychiatrists

THE VICIOUS CIRCLE IN COMPULSIVE DRUG USE

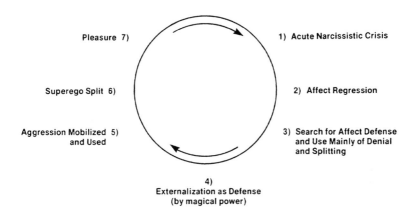

Pleasure 7)   1) Acute Narcissistic Crisis

Superego Split 6)   2) Affect Regression

Aggression Mobilized 5)   3) Search for Affect Defense
and Used   and Use Mainly of Denial
                                                  and Splitting

4)
Externalization as Defense
(by magical power)

and many psychoanalysts? Or to turn to the next objection: Are the internal and external structures and safeguards against these affects not often in many other people very brittle, just like the ground around a geyser: apparently firm, but breaking in at smallest weights and letting the boiling water flood over; is affect regression not a very common occurrence? And thus we can march down the list together and eliminate all distinctiveness. It appears to me, and I cannot be more than hypothetical, that the *combination is distinctive. Defective affect defense* (of those inner structures that channel affects, eventually becoming part of the predisposing personality structure), combines with the two most specific and most important factors: a) deep-going and *labile, rapidly shifting splits*, largely resulting from the *all-pervasive* use of the defense mechanism of *denial*, especially against affects, and b) the *massive defensive use of externalization* in its characteristic *concreteness of action*. This combination in its severity and massivity marks these patients and sets them apart from all others. This bold claim is based on a careful comparison in my mind of my toxicomanic patients with a number of neurotic patients having ostensibly somewhat similar problems whom I see in analysis, but who have never developed any drug problems. Whether this specification will hold up, however, only further comparative scrutiny will show.

Affect Regression and Breakdown of Affect Defense

This phenomenon which is shared by *all* toxicomanics and by many other borderline patients is also described as generalization, radicalization, totalization of affects, or, as Krystal and Raskin (1970) did, as dedifferentiation, resomatization, deverbalization. The terms are ponderous, the facts simple: The feelings become suddenly and irresistibly overwhelming, fearfully out of control. Words cannot do justice to them, nor can they be clearly differentiated from each other: Anxiety, anger, despair, pain etc.—all flow into each other. Henry Krystal (1974) devoted a special and excellent article to this concept, which had been developed by M. Schur (1953, 1966).

All compulsive drug users have the following affects in common, which have to be warded off by all means (not only by drugs). All these feelings are the direct outcome of narcissistic frustration. Some of them are more prevalent in one type of drug use, others in another form, but basically they are all there. These basic moods and affects are: *disappointment, disillusionment, rage, shame, loneliness and a panicky mixture of terror and despair.*

In a short survey we can glance at the correlation of specific affects denied, the nature of the narcissistic wish fulfillment attained, and the preference for certain types of drugs.

(a) The narcotics user has to cope with the emotional *pain and anxiety* flowing from the entire array of affects mentioned above. Among them *rage, shame and loneliness* seem particularly prominent. What he attains on the side of wish fulfillment is a sense of *protection, warmth and union*, of *heightened self-esteem and self-control.*

(b) The user of barbiturates and other sedatives has to deal with nearly the same task. Perhaps the feelings of *humiliation, shame and rage* are particularly prominent and need the most powerful form of denial: that contained in *estrangement* (partial or total depersonalization and derealization). Thus, a study of the barbiturate addict has to pay particular attention to that peculiar form of compromise formation; depersonalization is not simply a defense. Particular wish fulfillments are contained in this symptom and need to be studied in depth. (However, this does not mean that we shall not meet in most other toxicomanics hints of this very important symptom, although it is most prominent in the user of hypnotics.)

(c) In psychedelic users the major affects to be denied are the moods of *boredom, emptiness, lack of meaning;* from the primary list too, it is mostly *disillusionment and loneliness* which is walled off with the drug's help. What is attained—as gratification—is a sense of *meaning*, *of value*, *of admiration* and of *passive merger*—concerning the self as well as ideals.

(d) The users of stimulants, again beyond the primary list, fight against a particularly intense *form of depression, despair, sadness, loss. Shame about weakness and vulnerability, boredom and emptiness*, are quite prominent. The narcissistic gain lies in the feelings of *strength, victory, triumph, invincibility and invulnerability* that reaches in some nearly a manic state. The importance of *magical control*, ubiquitous in all categories, is particularly marked in this group.

(e) Alcoholics are less subject to the primary feelings listed above; the main feelings denied appear to be *guilt and loneliness*, also in many, shyness, shame, social isolation. The narcissistic gratification lies in the expression, not in the denial, of *anger* which had been so long suppressed or repressed. In many there is also the feeling of *company and togetherness*, of *shared regression* and *acceptance in a childlike status*, the overcoming of being an outcast, when alcoholized.

These manifold negative affects break through with unrestrained force when archaic narcissistic demands are thwarted. Many of them are already expressions of aggression, the twin brother of narcissism (cf. Freud 1930; Eissler 1971, 1975; Rochlin 1973). In the section on predisposition the connection of the two will be studied in a new light.

We have seriously to ask ourselves, however, whether this *radicalization and totalization* is simply a breakdown of deficient inner structures, of primitive defenses, or may be in itself a form of defense. Clinical experience with borderline characters (not solely compulsive drug users) leads me to presume that it can be both: manifestation of a structural defect as well as a defense.

This becomes clearer when we see how this *affect regression* leads to a regressive generalization of perception and cognition. It is the exaggeration of a correct perception, e.g., its *generalization* from one injustice and unfairness or hurt to the whole life. This *global* spread, like oil on water, I have often witnessed during sessions.

This affect regression is of central importance for the character structure of all patients with severe drug problems; and it is a totalization not restricted to some minor areas and choices; it permeates the whole world view for certain periods, until they can make it relative again. If they cannot do this, I think we deal with a *paranoid* deepening of the character pathology already outlined.

Very often it is experienced merely as a vague, but overwhelming physical *tension and restlessness*.

This entire phenomenon of affect regression is intertwined with a factor of the underlying personality, of the predisposition: the factor of *hyposymbolization*, the stunting of symbolic processes (for a brief note, cf. below). In regard to the question of compromise formation: All this stormy boiling up of affects is an outlet of regressed instinctual drives, mainly many forms of aggression. Simultaneously we have already remarked how this "totalization" serves as a defense, a flight from all too painful, all too limiting, crushing reality.

The Search for an Affect Defense

This third step is the most difficult to conceptualize. The patient is, as we saw, overwhelmed and flooded with unmanageable affects and often also most intense wishes, mostly destructive ones. His usual defenses have proven deficient. It is here that the drug enters —as memory or fantasy, then as sought-after means of solution, and finally as *found* help and protection, as a discovered coping mechanism (Khantzian et al. 1974).

When Dorian Gray recalled the murder of his (homosexual) admirer, mentor and father substitute, Basil Hallward, the morning after, he felt: "It was a thing to be driven out of the mind, to be drugged with poppies, to be strangled lest it might strangle one itself." Many observers have noted that all compulsive drug use is to be considered an *attempt at self-treatment*, and that the specific importance of the drug effect can be best explained as an *artificial or surrogate defense against overwhelming affects*, at least on a par with the aspect of wish fulfillment. Moreover it was already noted that there evidently exists some specificity in the choice of the drug for this purpose. But then the problems become so difficult and complex that one is tempted to exclaim with one of Dicken's characters: "'Tis a muddle, and that's aw." And yet it is perhaps the most crucial issue to be solved if we want to gain a deeper comprehension of compulsive drug use.

What is the nature of the defenses employed in these patients and propped up or instituted with the help of the pharmacological effect? The answer to this question is difficult and complicated.

When we examine the nature and order of defense "mechanisms," we should keep in mind what was briefly touched upon earlier—that the same processes we encounter as defense mechanisms can also serve as instinctual drive derivatives, as controlling processes of perception and cognition, and as basic action patterns (beyond drive-motivated ones). Moreover we can arrange them in several continua. These continua stretch from highly differentiated, subtle, usually mostly preconscious-conscious ones, to defenses operating on an archaic, undifferentiated level, functioning in a state of low integration, of global overinclusiveness, and, as processes, carried by a most peremptory, i.e., unconscious force. As to the latter I refer to Kubie's (1954) and Sandler's (1969) hypothesis: the more peremptory, compelling, rigid, inflexible, the more pushed by unconscious motivation (even if the process itself appears on the surface to be conscious).

Despite the current onslaught against the energy concept in psychoanalytic theory formation I find it, also in this context, a most useful, albeit metaphorical, one. The defenses on the more mature end of the continua operate with "neutralized," sublimated "energies," those toward the primitive end, are, even experientially, when analyzed, of quite archaic instinctual, mainly directly aggressive quality.

I suggest to consider these defenses as lying on four continua: a. A first continuum, the *avoidance type of defenses*, stretches from *conscious and preconscious proclamations* and wishes: "I do not want to know" (in Trunnell and Holt's paper: "denial" in the vernacular sense: "a 'declaring' not to be true") over *neurotic (unconscious) forms of denial* (keeping the affective significance of perceptions and entire parts of percepts unconscious) and *repression* (directed against drive derivatives) to very regressive, much more *global forms of denial* (of psychotic or near psychotic proportions).

This first continuum is artificially instituted or, far more likely, massively *reinforced by depressant drugs:* narcotics, hypnotics, minor sedatives and alcohol. The *other two types* (psychedelics and stimulants) sometimes support especially denial, sometimes *lift* these defenses; their major action lies, however, in what follows.

Amongst all these defenses lying on the continuum, conscious "disavowal" and *massive unconscious denial* are by far the most prominent—immediately prior to drug use and then part of the drug effect.

Cognitively we find, e.g., the averting of attention versus the focusing of attention.

b. The second continuum pertains to the *dissociation type of defenses*, the breaking of connections. It stretches again from conscious and preconscious versions, as described by Eissler (1959) and also in the Glossary (Moore and Fine 1968): *conscious isolation* in concentrated thinking, the *conscious ego split and superego split* in the psychoanalytic situation, to unconscious *isolation*, and the various forms of *splitting accompany-*

ing denial (denial of loss, of castration), to more regressive types (Kohut's "vertical" splitting and the limited, *partial forms of fragmentation*), and, beyond: to very severe, erratic, *labile* forms of *dissociation and pervasive splitting*, and to the two most extreme forms of *global splitting* into all-good and all-bad and of radical, *psychotic fragmentation.*

Dissociation's cognitive usefulness in concentration was commented upon by Freud (1926) and Eissler (1958).

In all compulsive drug users severe forms of splitting and fragmentation can be encountered. The *depressant* drugs usually *reduce* these dissociations and indeed thus help to synthesize, whereas particularly the *psychedelic drugs massively deepen the dissociation.* Whoever prefers splitting chooses psychedelic drugs.

c̲. The third continuum pertains to the *action or fight type of defenses:* again from conscious, controlled use (alloplastic change, creative use of externalization, outright aggression as defense) to unconscious *externalization*, turning *passive into active*, possibly even identification with the *attacker* and *reaction formation*, turning aggression *against the self*, and magical *undoing*, all on various levels of primitiveness. From all these, *archaic forms of externalization* will loom up as an omnipresent, massive form of defense in all compulsive drug users and will be treated separately. *Stimulants* are the one category of drugs which particularly *supports* the defenses on this continuum, especially *externalization and aggression, turning passive into active,* often in a very primitive form.

d̲. A fourth continuum of far more cognitive and action-oriented significance than for defenses is the continuum of the *boundary and limitation type of defenses*, stretching again from highly differentiated and preconscious forms of boundary forming and limit-setting "mechanisms," of boundary creation and breaking, to the most archaic forms of fusion, boundary and limit blurring and transgressing. Instinctually the continuum reaches from extreme merger to full separateness, cognitively from the archaic *syncretistic* thinking (Werner 1948) to full *differentiation and integration* (Hartmann, Kris, and Loewenstein 1946; Wynne and Singer 1963; also cf. Cassirer 1923), in action patterns in Piaget's sense, from "original reflex or global schemata" to schemata based on "generalizing assimilation" and differentiation (cf. Wolff 1960). In regard to the defenses on the one end we have largely preconscious identifying, learning and once again externalizing, also conscious detaching, separating and transgressing, whereas at the more primitive end we would encounter well-known archaic defenses like introjection and projection, radical idealizing and devaluing, primitive forms of externalization and identification.

I presume that the placing of one well-known defense "mechanism" (e.g., externalization) on several continua is quite justifiable, because the processes contained are often of multiple significance, and thus, multidetermining. I hold that in all drug abuse this fourth continuum of defenses (and beyond: of gratification, cognition and action) is used throughout and has particular importance. Since I presume that all four continua reach back into earliest childhood, I doubt whether any drug type by itself evokes a more or less regressive form of defense "mechanism" (and with that of conflict solution). Usually severity of preexisting pathology plus massivity of drug effect (usually dependent upon the dosage and the setting) determines the depth of regression on each of the four continua.

I do not pretend that I have encompassed all defense "mechanisms." It is quite conceivable that more forms and different lines can be found. It appears to me too that, as Hartmann postulated (Hartmann, Kris, and Loewenstein 1949), all defenses operate mostly with aggressive energies, often in very archaic, not "neutralized" versions. ". . . It is likely that defense against the drives (countercathexis) retains an element (fight) that allows of their description as being mostly fed by one mode of aggressive energy, and that this mode is not full neutralization" (1955, p. 232). This reference, including the indispensable energy metaphors, is amply demonstrated by the observations in drug patients: The pharmacogenic deepening of a defense is blatantly aggressive in nature, the pharmacogenic lifting unleashes overt conscious forms of aggressive defense (e.g., conscious disavowal and invalidation, use of direct violence for defensive purposes).

Thus the very deepening of the major defenses (denial, splitting, externalization) with the help of drugs is an act of destructive aggression, albeit intensely libidinous, especially narcissistic gains are also attained by the intensification of these defenses: the very muting of severely disruptive affects itself can lead to overwhelming feelings of joy, warmth, "good vibes" and, of course, as we will see in due course, much heightened self-esteem. Patients often become more sociable, friendly, accepting, harmonious, at peace, especially with depressant and psychedelic drugs.

This then leads to the conclusion that again this step, the pharmacogenic defense, is in truth a *compromise formation, in these patients, between their major affect defenses (denial, splitting, and externalization) and gratifications of aggression and libido,* in narcissistic and object related forms.

Splitting

When I use the term "splitting," I shall refer to it in three meanings, largely (though not fully concordant) with Lichtenberg and Slap's (1973) distinction: a) as disjunction and fragmentations of representations, b) in their extreme form as polarization into all-good and all-bad, and c) very importantly, as "splits" in the entire personality organization, what Schafer (1968), Lichtenberg and Slap called "pathological *intersystemic suborganizations*" or *"persistent drive-defense-prohibition couplings."*

Lichtenberg and Slap describe these couplings: ". . . manifestations of *defensive* activity become connected with a specific *drive* and with *superego* structures. . . . Associated with such drive-defense-prohibition couplings are elaborate networks of memories and displacements. These networks are built around the ideational contents of the developmental disturbance" (1973, p. 786).

Since these latter theoretical expositions are very abstract and difficult to understand, I try first to put them into somewhat simpler language: We observe in many, particularly borderline, patients a kind of "split personality."

In all forms I consider *splitting* a defense "mechanism" and the resultant *splits* experienced or observed as more complex phenomena, combining the *process* of splitting with hidden, unconscious gratifications, and filled with emotional and ideational *content.* When we now return to the three radical forms of splitting encountered in all compulsive drug users three features stand out: What I am most impressed with is the *lability* of these splits, the steady shifting of them, the *sudden flipflops.* Now there is synthesis—now there is a split. This pertains to feelings, to external limits, to self-image, the value of others, to ideals and to the conscience (cf. also Lucy Kirkman's test results [Wurmser 1977]). It is an utter unreliability of structures, an iridescence of denials and of experienced and often-described and observed "splits."

Secondly, these splits are very often covered over by depressants, exacerbated by stimulants and psychedelics. In the former instance (use of narcotics, hypnotics, alcohol) they become particularly evident during withdrawal and abstinence.

Thirdly, these splits always involve cognition. At the least it is what Freud described, the rending of the ego between two functions: e.g., the *acknowledgment* of the standing structures of the object world and the largely unconscious *disavowal* of such cognitive entities. Beyond this, in much broader terms, these splits profoundly affect the *cognition of objects and self, of time and space,* of all representations of self and object world, of one large part of the personality versus another massive part.

If we look back over what we have found, especially the prominence of denial and splitting, we are not surprised about the frequency with which these patients describe phenomena of depersonalization and derealization (see above). These twin symptoms occur either spontaneously or pharmacogenically. The more I study the material the stronger my suspicion becomes that if we only observe carefully enough we would find at least bits and pieces, if not the panoply, of the estrangement syndrome, in these patients.

Drug abuse thus seems like an artificial depersonalization state coupled with the next defense, externalization, which is so characteristic for "sociopaths."

Are drug abusers perhaps nosologically a *group uniting near psychotic estrangement with "sociopathy"*?

Externalization—The Neglected Defense

I set externalization apart, because it does not only function as a direct pharmacogenic affect defense (e.g., in stimulants, alcohol), but it has an overriding importance in *all* drug users in the form of seeking the solution to an inner problem on the *outside*, by *action* and in *concrete* form, quite apart from the eventually successful or failing function as affect defense.

This crucially important defense is the *action of taking magical, omnipotent control over the uncontrollable.* Everything else appears less specific compared with this peculiar and I think rather novel form of defense, valid for all compulsive drug taking. The anxiety is always there: "The various affects, like rage and depression, are going to overwhelm me." This fear of the traumatic state is powerfully warded off by the potent substance which is eaten, injected, snorted, or smoked: "I have the power—via this magical substance—to 'master' the rage, the pain, the boredom, etc." It is a specialized form of *defense by acting*—just as many analytic patients feel they solve an inner problem by an outer action (or avoidance of action), instead of by exploring, understanding and remembering. Moreover, since the Archimedean standpoint we have to take in psychoanalytic theorizing, after all, always addresses the inner stream of feelings and thought, any such act as utilizing an external help to "cope" with the frightening feeling, is a form of *externalization*—just like the picking of a fight by a guilt-laden patient or the carrying around of the powerful protecting lion by the boy who is afraid of his own aggression. Now all the rest falls into place too. Of course, one who *magically externalizes as a defense* against being overpowered by frightening affects uses the same defense in form of "concretization." He says, "It's not I who feels, it's society or the body which makes me suffer from this unnamable tension"—what was already referred to as *hyposymbolization*. One who thus externalizes by massive action cannot form the guiding values and ideals—again abstract, symbolic versions of early feelings toward persons. Instead the drug is a concrete, external, sought after vehicle of action. It stands in the place of the group of the most potent symbols: values and ideals—and the powerful drug effect replaces the power which values have for us, thus the chemical mythology!

Archaic guilt and shame are all over the place anyhow in these patients—the drug is both a magical protection, a *talisman* against them—from the outside—and an implementation of this *double Nemesis*—again from the outside. In other words: The drug tries to ward off externalized (mostly not yet internalized) retribution and humiliation, but simultaneously it functions itself as a punishment and as a shaming, a shameful proof of weakness and failure. The drug dependency is both a matter for boasting: the conquest of shame, and a cause for shame: an obvious weakness and failure, exposed for all to see, though anxiously hidden. The same interpretation holds for the *archaic dependency* and ties Kohut's and Anna Freud's view which seemed to contradict each other, together: the *defect in inner structures* lets the patient *seek an external object* of magical power to depend on for this all pervasive control. Again it is defense by externalization. *Externalization thus proves the magical key* for understanding not only all the proposed predispositions, but also so much of the external bluster. I have spoken sometimes—in connection with some cases—of the "Quadrangle of Fire" as a metaphor: All four "corners" are forms of externalization. It is the yearning for total unbound freedom, yet fatally abused; it is the need for security-lending structures, sought even as jail, but violently fought and rebelled against; it is the continuous search for adoration, the external confirmation of self-infatuation, the parading of phallic self-glorification; and it is the self-destruction by external means, the continuous arrangement of life that the patient has to flee like a hunted animal from police, mafia, vindictive whores —or imaginary enemies.

In contrast to paranoid states *the crucial "mechanism" of defense is not projection, it is externalization.*

And of course "society" falls in with it: "they"—police, politicians, physicians, parents, public (these five external powers)—go right along with the compulsive *drug user's demand for externalization:* They punish, prosecute, shame, hunt, prohibit, set up structures—inadvertently feeding this demand and becoming victims of it themselves.

In a sense the addict—like the paranoid—has been most successful in making the world serve his inner defense. Just as paranoid leaders influence world history by their terror-ridden projections, the addicts influence social history by their incessant demand for externalization. The success of both lies in forcing their surroundings near and far to play necessary roles in what is originally an internal conflict. The world goes along in this game of externalization, just as it does all too often with the projections of the totalitarian terrorists (whose concrete ideologies are but icing on their cake). These games of projection and externalization must have a potent lure for the "masses" to fall in so willingly.

But to return to the defense of externalization. That is surely not restricted to compulsive drug users? Do we not find it in many other patients (and nonpatients)? What then is specific for the form externalization assumes in the addicted person (even in its extensions—the TV addict, the gambler, the food addict, the compulsive smoker, the alcoholic)? It is the *magical* power invested *in a thing;* the *"thing" is endowed with control over the self,* over the inner life, over the feelings. The solution for any inner problem is sought in this one magical thing or type of things. The parallel case of endowing a *person* with such a magical power—very akin to the addictions—is the symbiotic surrender (and domination) in very regressed, often paranoid, but not necessarily psychotic patients. On the other, healthier side are those neurotics who externalize all over the place, but do not endow *one* thing (or type of things) with any of this exclusive magical power.

Kazin put this dynamic fact excellently: . . . "the addict to alcohol, like the addict to anything else, believes that he can *will* a change within himself by ingesting some material substance. Like so many of the things we do to ourselves in this pill-happy culture, drinking is a form of technology. . . . Drinking cuts the connections that keep us anxious" (1976, p. 45).

It is also blatantly obvious that externalization is thus not solely a defense mechanism, but also a wish fulfillment, above all the *wish for magical power,* the subcategory of narcissism stressed earlier—so again a *compromise formation.*

A few theoretical addenda to the concept of externalization (cf. Anna Freud [1965]) are in order here.
It is rather difficult to separate cleanly and clearly externalization from projection. The way I conceive the difference is that the emphasis in externalization as a defense lies on *action* (including and especially provocation), whereas in the case of projection as defense the emphasis is put on emotionally distorted *perception*. Obviously both often go hand in glove together.

We also can distinguish various modes of *defensive externalization:*

(a) by use of a *magically* powerful, mind altering, especially self-esteem increasing and affect-dampening *substance or thing;*

(b) by use of another *impersonal agent* as internal problem solver, like *television, gambling, money, food;*

(c) by use of an all-powerful, all-giving *personal agent* in *symbiotic* bonds or by fight against a *totally evil enemy* (here the projections are particularly prominent);

(d) by *lying*, manipulating and evading all personal commitments;

(e) by *transgressing* in grandiose "acting out" the limits set by nature and society (in what the Greeks called hubris, a specific characteristic of the "tragic character");

(f) by *provoking retaliation* in the form of shaming, of angry punishment or of diffuse attack;

(g) by outright *violence:* to destroy a symbolic representative of part of oneself, or, as in the just described mode, to bring about punishment;

(h) by *action as exciting risk*, especially if forbidden and dangerous, in an attempt to get rid of an almost somatic uneasiness and pressure, felt as primitive "discharge," a *breaking out of being closed in*, trapped, with undifferentiated but deeply frightening tension within. We saw how very typically the affect regression is experienced as a vague but broad, all-permeating *tension*, a drivenness and restlessness, a longing for risk and excitement. This tension is perhaps the prototype for all other modes of externalization.

In all these examples an external conflict situation and action ward off the internal conflict and the archaic overwhelming affects stemming from it. It is a very primitive group of defense modes. Also in all patients, this defense is combined with other defenses, above all—as we saw already—with splitting, regression and of course most massive denial, often with projection. All compulsive drug users show all or most of the eight modes of externalization described, concomitantly or alternatively.

As a general characteristic of all defensive externalization, we discern its *dehumanizing quality*. With the defensive use of action, this action itself is relevant, not the needs, qualities, properties of the persons "used," unless they happen to fit totally into this doing in the service of the denial. It is mainly this dehumanizing use of others which strikes us as so infuriating in all "sociopaths."

Another aspect of it has been described again by Eissler (1950): ". . . their tendency to accept only the concrete part of external reality as valid and valuable." He adds that "The tendency toward concreteness is mainly based on oral fixation and is also the result of the comparative deficiency in the ability to sublimate, which is significant of so many delinquents." This last remark, however, would lead us clearly into the question of predisposition and will be touched upon in that section.

But it is important that this fourth stage in our sequence is marked by the predominance of a magical, global form of externalization directed toward impersonal, concrete, dehumanized objects and action for action's sake.

An important aspect of externalization, in these patients at least, is so obvious that it is almost omitted. The defense of externalization reestablishes the illusion of *narcissistic power and control.* Most prominently in compulsive amphetamine users, but to an only slightly lesser extent in all toxicomanics we find fulfilled a *feverish wish for autonomy, for being in control,* an escape from the panicky fear of not being in charge of one's destiny, especially the most ominous "ghosts," the haunting representatives of one's inner life.

And since it is action, frenetic action, it always must *perforce use aggression in the service of this narcissism.* Externalization is obviously the exact opposite of inhibition: the blocking of the feared and wished action. Thus again this stage can be comprehended as a compromise formation.

Summary of the Direct Antecedents

When we summarize this section and repeat its main points we have to ask: "What is now the specific constellation, the final common pathway, immediately preceding acute beginning or resumption of compulsive drug use? What is essential and present every time?" It is the following group of indispensable phenomena:

(a) We noticed the externally precipitated, internally strongly experienced crisis in self-esteem, the severe narcissistic crisis, the collapse of expectations and valuations of the self and of others, and the reactivation of archaic narcissistic conflicts in an acute form. Their contents vary, from case to case, from time to time, appear isolated or in combination; but the acute precipitation of a conflict about self-esteem, valuation, meaning, in other words of an *acute narcissistic conflict* remains.

(b) This is followed by *affect regression*, a totalization and radicalization of feelings. The narcissistic conflict is either accompanied by *overwhelming feelings* of anger and rage, of shame and guilt, or boredom and emptiness, of loneliness and depression, or by a vague sense of wanting "excitement," adventure, to feel alive, oneself, awake, not estranged any more, a broad ill-defined tension, and sense of emptiness. This totalization serves at least partly defensive functions.

(c) The third component is the urgent, again acute, need to defend against these overflooding, overbearing affects—above all by *denial* and *dissociation;* these two are the major *affect defenses*, now *pharmacogenically supported*, because insufficient in their own right. They affect not solely the emotional life and the underlying instinctual drives, mobilized in the crisis (most prominently intense sado-masochistic impulses, often of uncontrollable intensity), but all of reality testing. It is an acute, pervasive, and characteristically varying, labile, but *very destructive ego split*. The splitting up may be of varied severity: in fetishism, a narrow one, or more extensive disjunctions and partial fragmentations or an overall polarization into all-good and all-bad. The combination of denial and splitting very often leads to typical states of depersonalization and derealization, with and without drugs.

(d) The fourth, most specific, most intense component is the use of *externalization* as defense: "I have to find an external solution for the unbearable internal problem which I do not want to see, cannot cope with, and yet am not able to avoid entirely either. I have several ways of external action: If I cannot find the *magical substance*, I choose one of the other avenues"—one of the other seven modes described. They are initially exchangeable and typically combined. The crux is: *action, "excitement," risk*—as a lightning rod for what is mobilized and denied.

(e) This defense by externalization carries intense *sado-masochistic* impulses with it; very often these aggressive intents are most vehemently repressed and denied, feared to the extreme, and yet palpably and indispensably present.

(f) There is not merely an ego split; there is a characteristic sudden "inoperativeness," a collapse of the superego, and an appearance of much more primitive forms of superego functions, a surprising, abrupt change from more mature, more integrated functioning of conscience, responsibility, ideals, to a much more primitive one, very often even a side-by-side existence of the two forms of superego. This superego with a suddenly unmasked Janus head is the *split in the superego*. This sixth constituent, ineluctable part of the specific cause, the *acute splitting of the superego*, occurs under the onslaught of the urge for externalization, for impetuous, impulsive, seemingly redeeming action.

(g) Finally, the end goal is getting "high" or at least finding relief—the euphoria, the regressive pleasure, usually of a combined narcissistic, oral, object-dependent nature, and, as part of the narcissistic fulfillment, a sense of being a cohesive, bounded self again. Furthermore, claustrophilia wins out over claustrophobia.

This is the *heptad of compulsive drug use*, which we have called the "vicious circle" and now described psychoanalytically as a series of complex compromise formations, appearing in this order, in this sequence, each dependent on its predecessor, a vicious circle of mutual reinforcement and malignancy.

SOME COMMENTS ABOUT PREDISPOSITION

We have described a perspective on a *horizontal* plane, which encompassed mainly a microanalysis of the structural, dynamic, topographic and some economic and adaptational factors as they are needed to understand the historically closest and logically most specific antecedents directly leading up to the addictive syndrome. We should add a *vertical* perspective—a look into the historical depth of the personality, an attempt to see the aforementioned factors in their genesis and unfolding.

Skepticism is particularly justified in our field. What Eissler (1969) wrote in regard to treatment holds true no less for theory:

Strangely enough, psychoanalysis is not able to provide the tools with which to combat the majority of forms in which drug addiction is now making its appearance among the younger generation in the United States. It seems that, just as psychoanalysis is, with few exceptions, not the method of choice in acute conditions, so it is not prepared to stem the tide of that form of psychopathology that is provoked by *anomie*. The dissolution of societal structures does not travel solely the path of lessening the strength of institutions and finally abolishing them entirely (at least for the time being), but also the path of *reducing structure in individuals*. The structure of the *ensuing psychopathology seems to be quite different* from the psychopathology whose treatment led to the evolvement of psychoanalysis (p. 463) (my italics).

Thus we face the following obstacles to a genetic exploration: (a) The methods of psychoanalytic inquiry have to be modified to such an extent in the treatment of these patients that the observations gained do not lend themselves easily to simple and minor modifications of the theoretical abstractions gained by the classical method.

(b) Very few patients stick to psychotherapy long enough to allow us sufficient genetic reconstructions which would give us the security of empirical probability.

(c) As Eissler noted there is such an intertwining of intrapsychic with familial, societal, cultural pathology that we cannot investigate and understand one without at least trying to do this for the others.

(d) The drug user himself is crippled by his very symptom in some of the core processes of judgment and self-recognition. Retrospective falsification is an ever-looming danger.

(e) The main tool of recognition in psychoanalysis, the transference neurosis, only most rarely becomes clear in treatment. The therapist has to assume so much of a reality role, the patient is so intolerant of deprivation, that very little indeed remains of the "as-if" nature needed to explore in a systematic way the transference aspects (Tarachow 1963)—no matter how hard a good, conscientious therapist and analyst tries to keep these parameters to a minimum. Very often the choice is between keeping the patient in treatment or even alive versus maintaining a therapeutic relationship allowing a maximum of theoretic insight.

In favor of our efforts are, however, a few clear insights:

(a) The heptad (see page 47) gives us plentiful clues to tie very many processes, seen in our patients as an ensemble, together with similar processes in other patients where they may appear "in single file."

(b) There is no question that most or all of these patients suffered very massive traumatization all through their childhood, mostly in the form of gross violence and crass seduction and indulgence. What neurotics show mainly as intrapsychic conflicts with preponderance of fantasy, these patients experienced as massive *external* conflicts of overwhelming dimensions from early childhood right through adolescence.

(c) Thus drug use is not simply an adolescent crisis gone awry (as the parents regularly want us to believe).

All compulsive drug users whom I ever got to know show what Kernberg so excellently described and studied as "borderline personality organization" (Kernberg 1967, 1970a and b, 1971, 1975). Here I stress mainly the predominance of primitive mechanisms of defense, i.e., of splitting, of primitive idealization, of early forms of projection ("projective identifications": "They have to attack and control the object before [as they fear] they themselves are attacked and destroyed"), of primitive manifestations of denial (" 'mutual denial' of two emotionally independent areas of consciousness"), and of omnipotence and devaluation. Kernberg also points to the lack of superego integration and easy reprojection of superego functions, the protective shallowness of their emotional relationships, their demandingness and exploitiveness, the chameleonlike quality of their adaptability and "as-if" quality.

But any such excerpt does injustice to the depth and richness of Kernberg's concepts.

Suffice it to note here that the toxicomanic patient allows us a detailed study of some of the traits shared by all "borderline" patients—especially splitting, denial and idealization (let alone the intolerance to anxiety and impulse, the blurring of ego boundaries), —but also permits us to gain rather novel insights into the role of manifold externalizations, the problems of affect tolerance and affect regression in general (not just anxiety), the important role of depersonalization, and especially the broad spectrum of various forms of boundaries and limits.

(d) As Eissler and Kohut in particular emphasized: These archaic personality organizations reflect a lack of inner structures which early damage and family and societal pathology conspire to bring about. A fourth aspect, usually omitted, may play a very important role in this lack of inner structures: heredity. How important a role, we have no way of knowing today, but this is a scientific problem open to experimental solution.

(e) The seven factors enumerated in the heptad all point to very archaic fixations—to problems in the first 2-3 years of life, to severe damage suffered at the time when these inner structures need to be built, when the child has to come to terms with frustrations to his omnipotence, to oral gratification, when boundaries between self and others are established, when he gradually learns to establish his own regulations of self-esteem, and, most importantly, when his affects become differentiated, put in symbols (including words, but not restricted to them) and slowly become manageable (cf. Schur 1953, 1966, especially Krystal 1974). There is no question that the severest damages in our patients lie in these early, largely preverbal times, though perpetuated on and on, as massive narcissistic conflicts and primitive aggressions directed with little differentiation against others and the self, as a general problem about boundaries and limitations, as archaic forms of defenses, as structural deficiencies of manifold nature.

Although we need particularly in this area far more specificity than our current theory provides us, I restrict myself to a cursory summary of the extensive findings presented in my full-length study.

If I try to select the one trait in the personality of the compulsive drug user which is most specific, it is the *overall lability of inner structures and of boundaries*. Not only are the emotions inconsistent and overwhelming, but so are the defenses, the self-other boundaries, generally the perceptual boundaries, and the limitations and boundaries watched over by the superego. Clinical experience, social and administrative observations and the test findings described especially by L. Kirkman (Wurmser 1977), all converge on that one point: the inner *"anomia,"* lawlessness, *the lack of consistency, structure, boundaries.* As Kohut so rightly remarks: This is the expression of a profound narcissistic defect. On the one side it is the outcome of acute and chronic narcissistic conflicts; therefore, the archaic, peculiarly narcissistic affects are overwhelming and unrestrained. But on the other side there is also a profound deficit *in structures* to cope in any consistent way, with the help of a reliable defense constellation, with such conflicts and ensuing affects. Withal we encounter this peculiar *shift of boundaries and limits of all sorts*, concretely and metaphorically.

The analysis regarding structure formation comes down to the cycle shown in the accompanying figure. One may separate the five elements into different defenses or defects; it is perhaps more accurate to view them as different parts of the same phenomenon which appear as defenses and as defects. When we look at it as denial, we emphasize the defensive aspect; when we stress splitting, we view the double nature of disavowal or denial and acceptance or acknowledgment, especially from a cognitive point of view; and finally when we focus on the boundaries, structures, and lack of effective affect defense, we seek mainly the "defect" nature of the phenomenon.

Again, as on the level of the immediate antecedents, we see the entire constellation of the predisposition as *necessary* preconditions. Among them I consider this element of an inner "anomia," this peculiar lability in structures, as the most specific one.

The pathogenic conflicts probably reach, as in schizophrenics, very far back: to *the most archaic conflicts in perception and expression* and, with that, to the original forming of any boundaries and self-nuclei. These conflicts are postulated to form a specific part of what is too loosely and broadly known as the oral stage.

The massivity of other (though closely related and overlapping) problems, especially of severe and archaic narcissistic conflicts in the patient and the gravity of inconsistency, aggression and promotion of externalization and deception in the family, are invariably present. These other necessary parts of the precondition are: hyposymbolization; labile, often externalized superego; defect in

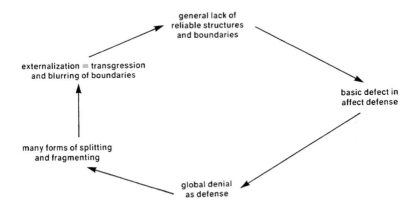

CYCLE OF STRUCTURE FORMATION
IN THE PERSONALITY OF THE COMPULSIVE DRUG USER

ideal and value formation; prevalence of shame; massive aggression, mainly of the rage and contempt type, more self-directed than against others (cf. Wurmser 1974).

Even in the predisposition of the patient himself usually the entire heptad described as the "final common pathway" can be discerned throughout life and becomes usually very prominent in adolescence.

If we compare this predisposition, the personality, the "set," with other nosological categories, the work with patients who are not compulsive drug users (e.g., psychoanalytic patients) allows a strong contradistinction: Above all, the intensity and archaic nature of narcissistic conflicts are usually much more pronounced in toxicomanics. The extent of boundary problems and the prevalence of the very archaic defenses of denial, splitting and externalization are most striking. Neurotics use, instead, much more repression, introjection, or the obsessional defenses. Projection appears in both to a moderate extent. The superego pathology is far deeper in addicts than in all types of neurosis. Finally, a strong case can be made that the peculiar form of aggression which is evident in shame, namely *contempt, disdain, scorn*, plus undifferentiated rage, but less anger and hatred, are the ones which are particularly prominently used in the service of externalization in these patients, and this even more in a self-directed, masochistic version, than against the outer world.

In contrast to the various psychoses the extent of ego split and superego split and, more generally, of fragmentation of cognition and perception is less strong in addicts. Projection, dehumanization, depersonalization are much stronger in psychotics during the acute phase than in addicts. Recompensated psychotics have much in common with recompensated addicts: If anything, the propensity to the characteristic splits, fragmentation, denial and externalization, even projection, the extent and massivity of narcissistic and sado-masochistic problems may even be more manifest and conspicuous in the addictive than the latently psychotic personality.

The theoretical conclusions presented here could serve us as a starting point to go in three directions—first, to systematic research of the hypotheses presented here, second, to a more thorough metapsychological exploration of these clinical observations, and third, to applications for prevention and treatment which would go beyond the present mad rush into action before thinking.

Research would have to proceed from this nodal point of the etiological equation in several directions. Of course, one road would lead simply toward *confirmation* (or refutation) and deepening of these findings. Another even less paved road would be a genetic exploration tying the described defects and conflicts together with developmental disturbances and family pathology. On another path, one would have to study the *constitutional* factors involved; at this point, we have no way of knowing how much of the underlying problems are of hereditary nature. Yet study beyond speculation is particularly tantalizing in this area. Still another route goes in an altogether different direction: The defects in ideal formation may open a deeper understanding for *value psychological* and value philosophical questions; thus such a study would assist us in a more thorough theoretical superego analysis than has been known hitherto.

TREATMENT

A few fragmentary thoughts about treatment need to be added, first, regarding psychotherapy and then regarding large-scale treatment policy.

Psychotherapy

One thing is clear above all: One cannot do "business as usual" with this type of patient. They resemble in many regards psychotic patients. Despite the usually dismal prognosis, I have seen a number of very severe chronic drug abusers successfully in long-term therapy. I think in particular of several patients who had been dependent for 10-20 years on very high doses of amphetamines (100 mg and more, or similar stimulants) or of narcotics (with dosages of 100-800 mg of methadone daily), whom I saw for one or several years. Looking back over these experiences, I single out one precondition of treatment which has facilitated successful treatment in several instances: the readiness on both sides for intensive, analytically oriented work and to stick it out no matter what. By "intensive" I mean often—in times of crises three to seven sessions a week, and sometimes much longer than 1 hour, plus telephone availability in times of lesser urgency. I have had cases who decompensated repeatedly and required brief hospitalizations (e.g., for suicidality in the case of amphetamine abstinence—often many months after withdrawal), but were able to work out their problems sufficiently in such very intensive psychotherapy that they were not only capable of assuming highly responsible positions, but eventually also to enter psychoanalysis proper. Given the severely regressive nature of the entire personality organization, it gradually became clear to me that the treatment situation has to encompass the following built-in transference elements:

(a) It has to have strongly *nurturing, supportive* elements without, however, feeding into the often overwhelming fears in the toxicomanic patient of *engulfment*. The therapist has to be far more *active*, warm, interested, personally involved, yet again without becoming *intrusive*, as very often the mother was.

(b) Also in all instances the exact counterpart has to be observed as well: to maintain *distance*, to be very patient, not pressuring, almost detached, without, however, supporting the profound sense of *abandonment and despair* so deep in these patients. One has to create a clear boundary of separateness, an atmosphere of nonsymbiosis and respect for individuality while still allowing symbiotic conflicts to be expressed and to become interpretable. The patient must not feel exploited and treated as a nonhuman object, no matter how much he may try to do that to the therapist.

Clinical experience appears to indicate that there may be indeed two basic types of compulsive drug users, one far more afraid of engulfment (a preponderantly *claustrophobic* type), the other fearing much more isolation and loneliness (in whom *claustrophilic* needs prevail).

In the first type the distance needs to be preserved far more and far longer for trust to arise, whereas in the second type far more direct support is needed, making up for a traumatic sense of object loss.

In most cases, though a delicate balance needs to be found somewhere in the middle, a constant empathetic weighing is required of whether more nurturing or more distance is needed at the given moment.

(c) *Limit setting*, external structure is absolutely crucial. Time and again the patient needs to be faced with the alternative of curtailing some particularly noxious form of acting out or of forfeiting any true benefit from therapy and even the gains already attained. Each time of such an intervention is a crisis for the therapy. The patient may concur and work on the intense anger this limit setting evokes, with additional gain in self-control and with that in the ability to observe himself and in the working alliance. Or he may bolt, revolt, vanish, seeing the therapist's guardianship of boundaries and limits as yet a new form of entrapment, of intrusion, of enclosure. Therefore such interventions have to be used very sparingly and without any moralistic implication: Transgression of ethical or of any other boundaries has to be treated strictly as a symptom with severe self-destructive potential, the compulsiveness of which is the sole concern, not its antisocial (or socially positive) valence.

(d) This leads naturally to problems of *countertransference*. Outrageous disregard of limits is often enacted precisely to *provoke rage*, punishment and scorn from the therapist and thus to reconfirm the *masochistic triumph:* "No one can ever be trusted. I am suffering again betrayal and degradation, and thus I prove the basic unworth of human relationships; I can rely only on my actions and on nonhuman substances."

Or in turn the therapist becomes a masochistic partner, forced by the ostentatious suffering of the patient into endless giving and giving-in, or into going along with and thus once again *indulging* the severest, most pernicious regressions.

Again the therapist has to find a golden mean: actively to set limits, but without anger, sadism, shaming, and vindictiveness, and yet to be very flexible, patient, always oriented not toward ethical values in a narrow sense, but toward the central psychoanalytic value outlined.

(e) This *demand for giving* and indulgence may in some cases be overwhelming, especially in massively spoiled or severely neglected patients. The transference-countertransference bind may turn into a *sado-masochistic nightmare*, a severe negative therapeutic reaction and hence into defeat: rage, pain, hopelessness alternate with insatiable demands. Here the *dilution* of the dyadic therapy relationship may save both treatment and life. In a number of cases the splitting up of the therapeutic approaches, e.g., into a combination of individual, family and group therapy, carried out by different therapists, proved far superior to individual psychotherapy alone. This is again an approach directly contravening the one-track mentality already criticized (cf. also E. Khantzian).

(f) Whereas the transference-countertransference constellation is a kind of perversion of intimacy, the next is a type of distancing which can reach extreme proportions. In many patients it may take a real *therapeutic moratorium* of months, even years, of passive drifting, boredom, interrupted treatment, apparent endless stagnation, of a deep gloom of despair and hopelessness in the patient, at times effectively transmitted to the therapist, until a solid basis of trust has grown to start therapy in earnest.

This *moratorium of passivity* might be necessary not just because of the deep fear of intimacy, of the claustrum and thus the devouring, englutting mother, but also (and connected with it) because of dread of murderous aggression unleashed in submission to the power of the stronger "other."

In order to tolerate such a lengthy moratorium the therapist has not only to be patient and rather at peace with his own narcissistic needs, but I believe it likely that he needs two additional traits: First, he has to see in the patient strongly *redeeming features*, e.g., in the case described (p. 43ff.), there was an intense feeling in me, through the years of despair: "What a waste of a capable, likeable, highly gifted, basically honest person!" In this feeling of *respect* and esteem for him, there was of course a lot of *hope*, which kept outweighing nearly always the massive despair. Second, the therapist has, as Freud stressed, to subordinate his therapeutic zeal to *scientific curiosity:* to understand and to help to understand must take precedence over the wish to heal, to mold according to one's own value priorities. To wait may mean to build up trust and to show caring; but then to step in and to set the right limits at the right moment (the "kairo's") may be critically important.

(g) The *working alliance* was defined by R. Greenson (1967) as "the relatively nonneurotic, rational rapport which the patient has with his analyst" (p. 192). I believe this concept to be equally applicable to the analytically oriented psychotherapy commonly chosen with these patients. In most instances these patients are too sick, too self-destructive, too demanding to leave much room for such rational cooperation. At first their attitude merely consists of a gut reaction: "I have suffered enough; I want to start anew. The price I paid in the past I am not willing to pay in the future." Thus, it is not so much the value of rationality which attracts them, but the *fear of further pain* and suffering which pushes them from behind. But as the time passes (again often years) an *identification* with the value of inner freedom, of self-mastery, of non-condemning exploration and knowledge, as represented by the therapist, may replace the more archaic ego ideals, and gradually lend more and more force to rationality and thus to the working alliance. Hence, shame and guilt may become associated with such a standard of reason instead of the grandiose self-image which had ruled supreme.

Large-Scale Treatment Policy

Heavy (compulsive) drug use is *coextensive with moderate to severe psychopathology underlying the drug use, not caused by it.* The crisis in the treatment of these patients who are either rejected or inadequately treated by the currently existing programs is also *coextensive with the crisis in the treatment of* emotionally disturbed or outright mentally ill patients in general. Innovative facilities should be created employing the gamut of already known psychiatric techniques to this class of patients; it appears imperative to develop and implement *innovative psychotherapeutic techniques* specifically for this type of pathology—combining in-depth dynamic (psychoanalytic) understanding and leadership, structure building and limit setting, family treatment, vocational retraining (or new training), opening up of creative or recreational avenues of gratification, and the flexible use of psychopharmacological agents. In other words: *Instead of one-track modalities* we need *combinations* of four to seven methods for each individual patient in a methodical, specific way.

Such a plan calls for the *avoidance* of many of the current faddish "short-cuts" and fashionable new "simplistic" techniques, because of their destructive potential with these severely ill patients. It requests a deeper involvement in the positions of *leadership* by psychiatrists and psychoanalysts in dealing with the majority of the problems of compulsive drug use. The current debunking of a thorough training in psychiatry and especially in *intensive individual psychotherapy*, and with that the nearly *total lack of understanding for the psychodynamics of these patients and their families* has been devastating for psychiatry in general; but it has left the field of treatment of these patients almost entirely to paraprofessionals and to specialists from other fields who are naive as to the gravity and nature of the psychopathology in the majority of these cases and as to measures for devising rational treatment strategies for each individual case.

Most specifically, it calls for a *deeper involvement of psychoanalysis in such a leadership role*, not as a treatment method, but as the only accredited institution which has set itself the goals of a deeper systematic understanding of the human mind and of a methodical, thorough, well-structured and supervised training of its practitioners. Despite its current external and even internal crisis, its factual contribution to the huge problem at hand could perhaps be the *most innovative suggestion* this report can make—as old fashioned as it may sound to many readers.

Reluctantly, I have to break off. What I have presented is, naturally, condensed, fragmentary, but I believe it may give some hints whither the new developments evolving from intensive therapy have led us so far and may point onward.

To finish, suffice it to say that we cannot remain, in this field which often appears to me beset by ponderous rhetoric and fatuous motion, like Mr. Pecksniff's horse (in Dickens' *Martin Chuzzlewit*), ". . . full of promise, but of no performance. He was always, in a manner, going to go, and never going."

REFERENCES

Cassirer, E. *Philosophie der Symbolischen Formen* (1923). Darmstadt: Wiss. Buchges, 1958.
Eissler, K.R. Ego-psychological implications of the psychoanlaytic treatment of delinquents. *Psychoanal Study Child*, 5:97-121,1950.
———. On isolation. *Psychoanal Study Child*, 14:29-60, 1959.
———. Irreverent remarks about the present and the future of psychoanalysis. *Int J Psychoanal*, 50:461-471, 1969.
———. Death drive, ambivalence, and narcissism. *Psychoanal Study Child*, 26:25-78, 1971.
———. The fall of man. *Idem*, 30:589-646, 1975.
Freud, A. Normality and pathology in childhood. In: *The Writings of A. Freud*, New York: Int. Univ. Press, Vol. 6, 1965.
Freud, S. *Inhibitions, Symptoms and Anxiety* (1926). SE. XX. London: Hogarth Press, 1959. pp. 75-174.
———. *Civilization and Its Discontents* (1930). SE. XXI, London: Hogarth Press, 1961. pp. 57-145.
Greenson, R.R. *The Technique and Practice of Psychoanalysis.* New York: Int. Univ. Press, 1967.
Hartmann, H. Notes on the theory of sublimation (1955). *Essays on Ego Psychology.* New York: Int. Univ. Press, 1964, pp. 215-240.
Hartmann, H., Kris, E., and Loewenstein, R.M. Comments on the formation of psychic structure. *Psychoanal Study Child*, 2:11-38, 1946.
———. Notes on the theory of aggression. id. 3/4:9-36, 1949.

Kazin, A. "The Giant Killer": Drink and the American Writer. *Commentary*, 61:44-50, 1976.

Kernberg, O.F. Borderline Personality Organization, *J Am Psychoanal Assoc*, 15(3):641-685, 1967.

_____. Factors in the Psychoanalytic Treatment of Narcissistic Personalities. *J Am Psychoanal Assoc*, 18(1):51-85, 1970.

_____. A Psychoanalytic Classification of Character Pathology. *J Am Psychoanal Assoc*, 18(4):800-822, 1970.

_____. Prognostic Considerations Regarding Borderline Personality Organization. *J Am Psychoanal Assoc*, 19(4):595-635, 1971.

_____. *Borderline Conditions and Pathological Narcissism*. New York: Jason Aronson, 1975.

Khantzian, E.J., Mack, J.E., and Schatzberg, A.F. Heroin use as an attempt to cope: Clin. obser., *Am J Psychiatry*, 131:160-164, 1974.

Krystal, U. The genetic development of affects and affect regression. *Ann Psychoanal*, 2:93-126, 1974.

Krystal, H., and Raskin, H.A. *Drug Dependence. Aspects of Ego Functions*. Wayne State Univ. Press, 1970.

Kubie, L.S. The fundamental nature of the distinction between normality and neurosis. *Psychoanal Q*, 23:167-204, 1954.

Lichtenberg, J.D., and Slap, J.W. Notes on the concept of splitting and the defense mechanism of the splitting of representations. *J Am Psychoanal Assoc*, 21:772-787, 1973.

Moore, B.E., and Fine, B.D. *Glossary of Psychoanalytic Terms and Concepts*. New York: Amer. Psychoanal. Assoc., 1968.

Rado, S. The psychoanalysis of pharmacothymia (drug addiction). *Psychoanal Q*, 2:1-23, 1933.

Rochlin, G. *Man's Aggression. The Defense of the Self*. Boston: Gambil, 1973.

Sandler, J., and Joffe, W.G. Towards a Basic Psychoanalytic Model. *Int J Psychoanal*, 50:79-90, 1969.

Schafer, R. *Aspects of Internalization*. New York: Int. Univ. Press, 1968.

Schur, M. The Ego in Anxiety. In: *Drives, Affects, Behavior*. New York: Int. Univ. Press, 1953. pp. 67-100.

_____. *The Id and the Regulatory Principles of Mental Functioning*. New York: Int. Univ. Press, 1966.

Szasz, T.S. The problem of psychiatric nosology. *Am J Psychiatry*, 114:405, 1957.

Tarachow, S. *An Introduction to Psychotherapy*. New York: Int Univ. Press, 1963.

Trunnell, E.E., and Holt, W.E. The concept of denial or disavowal. *J Am Psychoanal Assoc*, 22:769-784, 1974.

Werner, H. *Comparative Psychology of Mental Development*. New York: Int. Univ. Press, 1948.

Wolff, P.H. Psychol. Issues. No. 5 *The Developmental Psychologies of Jean Piaget and Psychoanalysis*. New York: Int. Univ. Press, 1960.

Wurmser, L. Psychoanalytic considerations of the etiology of compulsive drug use. *J Am Psychoanal Assoc*, 32:820-843, 1974.

_____. *The Hidden Dimension: Psychopathology of Compulsive Drug Use*. New York: Jason Aronson, in press.

Wynne, L.C., and Singer, M.T. Thought disorder and family relations of schizophrenics. *Arch Gen Psychiatry*, 9:191-206, 1963.

CHAPTER 5

Substance Abuse: An Understanding From Psychoanalytic Developmental and Learning Perspectives

Stanley I. Greenspan, M.D.

The problem of substance abuse in any one individual must be understood in terms of the multiple lines of his development. It is not enough to simply view the substance abuse as a means of acting out an unconscious conflict with authority, or dealing with an underlying deep depression, or as part of a chronic antisocial character pattern. For any given individual, all, or none of these, might be contributors. Instead, in studying the problem of substance abuse, a model is needed within which the personality can be viewed from multiple perspectives at once. This is consistent with the psychoanalytic principle of multiple determination. According to this thesis, all behavior is a product of multiple determinants, e.g., unconscious and conscious, as well as genetic, adaptational, structural, and dynamic. Thus, for a given individual, using an addictive drug might incorporate at the same time, the satisfaction of certain primitive impulses and needs, a structural defect in one of the ego's substructures dealing with impulse or affect regulation, and an adaptation to an extraordinarily stressful environment.

Just two perspectives that the psychoanalytic model brings to understanding problems of substance abuse will be considered to illustrate the principle of multiple determination and the problem of drug addiction. The first is a developmental perspective; the second, an extension of the adaptational point of view, is a psychoanalytic learning model.

What follows will highlight some aspects of the developmental view of substance abuse so as to illustrate how different levels of development may contribute to a complex behavioral pattern. Though couched in terms of male development, the analysis is general enough and should be understood as applying as well to female development. First, consider that the infant attempts to reach a state of homeostatic peacefulness. He brings with him into the world a number of basic rhythms which help him achieve this. His environment helps to protect him from overstimulation and provides the physical and emotional nurturance necessary for him to obtain these peaceful homeostatic states. During this early period, in the context of a responsive and supportive maternal object, the infant begins his important task of attachment. He begins the first step in developing his uniquely human relationships. At the same time, his primitive impulses are beginning to organize around orality as a means of engaging the environment and achieving pleasure. His ego structure is beginning to attain some initial capacities for regulating his internal experience and finding effective ways of relating to his primary maternal figure and the inanimate aspects of his environment.

However, should either innate constitutional characteristics or a chronically severe traumatic environment hamper him in attaining these initial steps in his development, the infant may suffer severe deviations. For example, failure to attain the capacity to achieve regulation or homeostatic balance in the context of an attachment to a maternal object could be one determinant, among others, of later substance abuse. It is not uncommon to hear a substance abuser talk about the need to obtain the most basic and primitive kind of homeostatic experience. Often, this kind of basic stability in his internal world seems to be what is lacking. The substance, be it heroin or some other narcotic or stimulant, works at a physiologic and psychological representational level to facilitate the attainment of this basic homeostatic experience. Here, therefore, we can see a derivative of substance abuse behavior emanating from a very early period in an infant's life, even before the basic attachment to the maternal object.

Developmental deviations will occur if an infant does not achieve the basic capacity for attaching to a human object for a variety of reasons, e.g., unusual constitutional sensitivities on the infant's part; or a lack of availability of a pleasurable maternal object; or characteristics unique to the interaction of the infant with his primary maternal object. Substance abuse could emanate from the lack of this basic ability of attaching to the human object. In essence, substance abuse can become a substitute for this attachment. For some individuals basic attachments of this kind are possible only under the influence of drugs.

If an infant does obtain the developmental accomplishments needed to establish an emotional investment and attachment to a primary maternal object, he next discovers whether it is possible to get his needs met in the context of this human relationship. It is in this context that the infant also learns, through feedback from the maternal object, to experience aspects of his own internal world. Even basic states such as hunger become, in part, recognized by the infant through the responses his hunger elicits from the environment. Initially, it is feedback from the environment that allows the infant to understand the "means-ends relationships" within his own body. If certain internal feeling states, expressed by the infant, lead to certain predictable results in the environment, there is a consolidation of these early cognitive and affective schemes. It is not difficult to see how substance abuse at a later time could derive from a disturbance in the normal development of these early schemes. Hilde Bruch (1973), in her work with anorexia and overeating, has hypothesized a basic defect in the ability to experience internal feeling states such as hunger. Thus, anorexic people eat or do not eat because of external forces that are removed from the internal need state. In clinical interviews, many substance abusers speak not just of a sense of depression or deep internal pain, but of an anhedonic experience of feeling nothing inside; only a drug experience gives them an internal feeling state. This could be related to early experiences where the preliminary psychological structures necessary for experiencing organized feeling states are not constructed, due to an impairment in the early infant-mother interaction patterns.

As the infant moves toward the end of his first year, he should be beginning to consolidate a separate image of his "self" from the image of the primary objects around him. One could hypothesize how an inability to fully consolidate the self-other boundary could lead to the overwhelming anxieties often associated with later substance abuse. In this instance, the ingestion of addictive substances serves to consolidate for the individual an organized nonaversive sense of self, whether artificially induced by a drug "high" or "low."

If development thus far has been successful and an adequate attachment has formed between the infant and the primary maternal object, the task of separation and individuation then becomes crucial. While the infant, early in his second year of life, is demonstrating his increased motor coordination by crawling, walking, and running from room to room, we often note that he returns to his mother or other primary objects for "refueling." In this phase, he shows curiosity and takes delight in his environment. According to Mahler (1971), he is acting under the all-encompassing umbrella of parental omnipotence. During this stage, the infant can achieve an important sense of mastery. If, for example, this is interfered with because of a mother who needs to hold the infant too close, who is frightened of permitting the separation process to occur, the consolidation of the sense of mastery and the delineation of the infant's picture of himself as a separate being from his primary objects may suffer severe impairment. Because all this is occurring during a period of rapid growth in motor coordination, the infant has greater capacities to experience and channel aggressive feelings. At the same time, toward the middle and latter part of the second year, the infant's instinctual organization is beginning to organize around the mental representations concerned with anality. It is quite possible during this period, therefore, for interferences in optimal development to result in personality organizations that are either extremely passive, extremely negativistic, hostile and belligerent, or extraordinarily impulsive (almost as though to burst out of mother's grasp). Underlying all these personality organizations may be the primary impairment of an internal sense of mastery and delineation of self from the primary other. The use of drugs in an effort to obtain this primary, never acquired state of mastery and the clear demarcation of self that accompanies it, is also seen in clinical interviews with many substance abusers. The conflict during this developmental stage when the infant is at once merged with the parental omnipotence, but at the same time needs the freedom to explore his world, is also seen in those substance abusers for whom the underlying dynamic is related to unresolved issues of merging and separation. The substance becomes a way of obtaining a sense of oceanic merging with the omnipotent object and, at the same time, is safe enough, since it is a drug and not the omnipotent object. The user is not afraid of being literally "swallowed up."

If, in the context of a supportive family environment, the infant succeeeds in achieving the sense of mastery associated with the 12-to-18 month period of life, his maturational progress in the cognitive sphere permits him further to perceive his own "self" as distinct from others and to realize a sense of his own size in relation to his parental figures. For the first time the infant sees that indeed he is not a part of his mother, but rather, that he is totally separate and quite small. This can be very frightening. Margaret Mahler (1968) points out that it is during this "rapprochement" phase of development that the infant often returns to the primary maternal objects for further dependency support, going through another gradual separation process and emerging optimally into what Mahler refers to as the "libidinal object constancy" stage. According to Piaget (1952), with his growing capacity for "figurative thinking," that is for mental representation, the toddler can now have a picture of himself and his environment that is relatively more realistic than was possible for him at an earlier phase of his life. This capacity for mental representation places a new burden on him. Piaget (1952) and Mahler (1968) both agree that the infant and young child now repeat many of the steps that occurred earlier in development as they re-work issues at a higher level of mental representation than were first achieved at the level of acting on the environment. If the mother and/or others are not available to give the extra needed supports during this "rapprochement" phase, the child may experience tremendous anxiety, resulting in possible personality distortions.

Difficulties stemming from this crucial phase of development might, for example, center around a precocious sense of independence superimposed on a precarious, somewhat fragmented self-representation. Severe impairments in self-esteem and depressive constellations may develop. Because of the increased capacity for organized aggressive behavior and ego differentiation which accompanies the capacity for figurative thinking, a variety of defensive organizations may become manifest, such as impulsive acting out, depression, psychosomatic difficulties, and severe antisocial behavior patterns.

All of these can accompany underlying masochistic personality organizations consistent with the anal phase of instinctual organization. It is not surprising that we see a strong masochistic component in many severe characterologically resistant substance abusers, where the abuser is at one and the same time hurting himself and an internalized loved/hated object. Such behavior may very well emanate, in part, from this developmental period where the depended-upon object may have been perceived in a strikingly ambivalent way. At the very time it was the only available hope for dependency satisfaction, it was also the source of tremendous torture and suffering, since it did not fulfill these expectations of satisfaction. Thus, we can see how the substance that is being abused can serve multiple functions simultaneously. It can represent the ambivalently regarded object; it can provide the state of satisfaction sought after; and it can provide the outlet for the sadistic and masochistic components of unresolved rage.

As the young child moves toward the third year of life, it becomes possible for him to obtain true libidinal object constancy; that is, it becomes possible for him to retain a constant internal image of himself and important others. He can construct a constant, delineated boundary between those organized representations of himself and others which provides the foundation for differentiated ego structure and the ego functions, such as reality testing, impulse regulation, and synthesis of different internal and external experiences. This is occurring in the context of an instinctual organization shifting from anality to phallic concerns. In order for object constancy to be consolidated, however, the child must first be capable of experiencing mourning. To become capable of greater independent functioning, he must relinquish his dependent attachment to the real primary maternal object and go through a mourning period. If he is successful, he can then move into the phallic Oedipal stage proper, with a solid, differentiated ego structure to help him contend with the vicissitudes of drive and object relationships consistent with this new phase of development. Many youngsters, however, because of unresolved earlier issues, or because of familial circumstances, are not able to experience mourning and consolidate the internal representation of themselves and important others, and thus do not completely attain the stage of libidinal object constancy. Instead of letting go through experiencing sadness and mourning, they cling to the dyadic partner and defend against anticipated sadness and depression.

Substance abuse problems derived from this developmental phase often manifest themselves in the context of a fairly well organized character structure, although one which is incapable of feeling sadness or depression. Often, acting out and other antisocial defenses are then used as a way of attaining a kind of pseudophallic exhibitionism in the service of defending against underlying feelings of sadness and depression which have never been consciously experienced. The substance abuse, in this sense, is a defense against separation anxiety and its accompanying depression. Patients with difficulties stemming from this developmental stage, in long-term therapy may eventually talk about the fragility and tenuousness of their sense of self and/or others. Their concerns are heightened when they experience strong feelings such as anger, or during periods of separation. The patterns of substance abuse associated with this developmental period may be more intermittent and partially exacerbated by certain feeling states or experiences such as separation or loss.

If development has successfully emerged from this period of libidinal object constancy, the next major developmental task is to move into the triangular relationship patterns and the phallic Oedipal period proper. During this period, ages 3½ to about 6, the youngster becomes capable of organizing his personality in the context of a differentiated ego structure. All earlier conflicts and developmental interferences become organized in the "infantile neurosis." The infantile neurosis, in this sense, is an organizing structure which brings together all that has preceded it in the most economic fashion possible. The young child is now capable, for the first time, not only of internalized conflict, but of organized conflictual structures which, on the one hand, may be the precursors to later neuroses, but on the other hand, are an important developmental accomplishment. The personality achieves a certain cohesion, organization and structure which permits it to tolerate a wide range of internal and external experiences. A person who has achieved this stage has a relatively greater adaptive capacity than one who is fixated at an earlier developmental stage.

Individuals who have achieved this developmental level do not often manifest severe substance abuse problems. They tend rather to manifest organized neurotic and mild characterologic problems. However, if the neurotic structure is sufficiently incapacitating, substance abuse can be one way of diminishing anxiety. The substance abuse pattern may contain elements of unresolved Oedipal conflicts in both the positive and negative Oedipal organizations, as well as regressive preoedipal constellations either in isolation or as part of a consolidated neurotic structure.

Thus far, the relationship of different levels of the development of substance abuse patterns has been considered separately. In real life, of course, one may see a clustering of problems from many of these levels. An individual may deal adequately, if not optimally, with one stage of development and bring residual problems from that stage to a subsequent stage where there are additional problems. Thus, behavioral patterns become organized around multiple determinants from multiple developmental levels.

In addition, however, to have a complete understanding of any behavioral pattern, one must also consider dynamic, structural, and adaptive components of that pattern. While these additional determinants will not be dealt with at this time, they are also important.

PSYCHOANALYTIC LEARNING PERSPECTIVE

There is an additional perspective that combines elements of the psychoanalytic model with the operant learning model. In considering the problems of substance abuse, it is particularly important to enhance the existing perspectives already considered by psychoanalytic psychology with the *psychoanalytic learning perspective*. The theoretical base for a psychoanalytic learning perspective was developed in an earlier work (Greenspan 1975). The model derived from that work will be used for this discussion. The learning perspective forcuses on how certain features of environmental experience impact on the ego to influence behavior. The psychoanalytic learning model is unique in that it defines external experience in terms of classes of discriminative stimuli and reinforcers which are derived from stage-specific organizations of the ego and drives. For example, a substance abuser who achieves a basic and primitive homeostatic experience by using his addictive drug may be obtaining tremendous and potent reinforcement from the substance abuse. Reinforcers found in the environment may be undifferentiated and, therefore, of multiple types and found in multiple places. They may be defined as homeostatic-producing reinforcers. Not only drugs, but, for example, certain states of consciousness, or certain interaction patterns with important persons, may produce the homeostatic experience. Once a class of reinforcers functions as "homeostatic-producing reinforcers," the way in which this class of reinforcers operates instrumentally on the organized behavior patterns derived from the properties of drive and ego organization may play an important role in shaping substance abuse behavior and in making it more or less resistant to change. For example, it is well known that behavior under the influence of random schedules of reinforcement is relatively more resistant to change than behavior under the influence of continuous schedules of reinforcement. A substance abuser who uses drugs to achieve a "pleasurable high" only occasionally may be more difficult to wean from the drug than an abuser who uses drugs to achieve a "high" continually. While it is not possible to go into detail here about learning theory, it is important to note that learning theory extends our understanding of how the environment influences, shapes and modifies behavior in ways that are not at all obvious to "commonsense." It becomes especially important to have a learning perspective when dealing with an individual whose development has been arrested before he was able to fully internalize conflict and form integrated internalized structures. A person with an undifferentiated drive organization and a relatively undifferentiated ego structure experiences his environment with multiple peremptory needs and wishes, along with basic feeling states of incompleteness. Because of a lack of internalized control and the number of potent internal forces working from within, he tends to be vulnerable to environmental influences in rather dramatic ways and is sensitive to many potentially reinforcing events in his external environment. His behavior is more easily molded by external forces than the behavior of an individual who has achieved a higher level of personality integration. The reinforcing properties of the environment must therefore be considered as *another* determinant of behavior alongside the multiple determinants that have already been considered.

In addition to the developmental determinants already described, and the structural, dynamic, and adaptive determinants only alluded to, we must also consider learning determinants. We must understand the environmental determinants that have rather specific effects, depending on the structure and character of personality organization. The psychoanalytic learning model referred to earlier can help us understand the effects of environmental stimuli on the organization and maintenance of maladaptive patterns of behavior.

The learning perspective can be especially important as we design and set up treatment programs. We know from past experience that helping the substance abuser to reach a greater understanding of internal experience, including broadening his capacity for experiencing a wide range of internal ideas and feeling states may not be sufficient treatment. Often, the abuser acts out, or leaves treatment before he can be helped to reach a state of internalized regulation and self-esteem maintenance. To help a substance abuser stay in the treatment relationship so that psychological growth may occur requires an intricate understanding of how the external environment is interacting with his internal personality organization.

AN INTEGRATED MODEL TO UNDERSTAND
SUBSTANCE ABUSE PATTERNS

One approach to understanding patterns of substance abuse is in the context of a broad understanding of personality organization and its relationship to the organization of the environment. Along these lines, we might develop a grid designed to consider a number of aspects of personality functioning and related environmental factors in a developmental context. This grid might depict, starting at the top left corner, the level of drive organization; next, the organization of affects; next, the organization of internalized object relationships; next, the level and style of ego differentiation; next, the relationship patterns the person has achieved in the external world; and next, the organization of the person's external reality including the availability, patterns, and schedules of potent discriminative events and reinforcers. If these different categories were placed horizontally at the top of the grid, and the developmental phases from infancy to adulthood placed vertically at the left-hand side of the grid, we could then trace where the individual was at in a developmental context. Such a pictorial presentation might help us to understand better the pattern of substance abuse in the context of multiple aspects of personality functioning. Type of drug, pattern of use, accompanying psychopathology as well as strengths might be related to certain personality characteristics.

To be able to arrive at a comprehensive personality assessment and to understand the complexities of types and patterns of substance abuse requires, at the practical level, some personality assessment scales. These scales would permit people engaged in working with substance abusers to begin thinking systematically about this very difficult group of patients. To this end, reference should be made to some existing ego assessment scales, including those by Bellak (1964), and Greenspan and Cullander (1973).

The appendix of this paper contains a few items from the Greenspan and Cullander profile which may be used as a beginning in an attempt to define more systematically some of the personality characteristics which contribute to the type and patterns of substance abuse. It should be noted that this is only a beginning and conceptualizes only a few lines of personality organization. Items chosen from the profile were those that are relatively easy to score and are tied most closely to observable behavior. The items in the appendix are by no means a complete inventory, but represent a kind of screening of certain ego functions at a general level. It is hoped that this will begin the process of systematic assessment of all substance abusers in order to understand better their similarities and differences.

APPENDIX[1]

1. Ego intactness (vs. ego defects)
Included in this category is the general basic integrity of the ego in terms of an evaluation of the ego apparatuses and functions.

(a) Ego Apparatus—This category includes the basic organic integrity of the ego: for example, the perceptual apparatuses (visual, auditory), the motor apparatuses, apparatuses that coordinate these (perceptual-motor), and other similar apparatuses, such as memory, that have to do with the integrity of the mental apparatus.

(b) Basic ego functions—This category should include only the basic overall functions of the ego (reality testing, predominance of secondary-process thinking, presence of ego boundaries). Special attention should be paid to the more subtle aspects of these functions that will give the interviewer clues about well-hidden borderline organizations; for example, preponderance of magical thinking,

---

[1]Reprinted with the permission of International Universities Press, Inc., from the *Journal of the American Psychoanalytic Association*, Vol. 21, No. 2, 1973.

diffuse thinking, facile rationalization, extreme naivete, or action orientation covering up ego defect.

Good
The organic ego apparatuses and basic ego functions are basically intact. Interference from neurotic formations are minimal to none.

Fair
Either physical or psychological factors (neurological dysfunction, functional ego defects, characterologic constrictions) *moderately* impair the ego's capacity.

Marginal
Same as above except they *markedly* interfere with ego's capacity.

Inadequate
Either physical or psychological factors *severely* interfere with the ego's capacity (severe neurologic dysfunction, ego defects resulting in psychotic processes, etc.).

2. Ego flexibility (vs. rigidity)
This category assesses the flexibility of the ego in its capacity to utilize a variety of finely discriminated operations, in contrast to the degree to which the ego is rigid, with only a few poorly discriminated operations at its disposal. Included are the capacities to form and tolerate internal conflict and a variety of appropriate affects as compared with signs of arrested ego development, ego constrictions (severe character disorders), externalization of conflict, and altered or restricted modes of drive gratification (perversion). In addition, symptom formation which does not grossly interfere with ego functioning should be contrasted with symptoms or affects which lead to a breakdown in ego functions or further constrictions (withdrawal).

Good
The ego is relatively flexible in its response to internal or external stimuli. Neurotic formations only minimally interfere with this flexibility.

Fair
The ego is somewhat rigid, but along with these ego constrictions is a capacity to tolerate internal conflicts without marked disruptions in ego functioning (mixed characterologic and neurotic difficulties).

Marginal

The ego tends to be rigid in its operations. Neurotic formations *markedly* intensify this rigidity and/or lead to minimal breakdowns in ego functioning such as temporary losses of reality testing, loss of sense of self, temporary loss of capacity to integrate thought and affect, severe states of inhibition, or alteration of drive gratification

Inadequate

The ego uses severe constrictions and only a few poorly discriminated operations (defenses) to cover more basic structural defects, (as seen in psychotic or borderline organization).

3. *Affects (multiple, flexible, developmentally advanced vs. few, rigid, developmentally retarded)*

This category should include an assessment of:

(a) The types of affects (those that predominate and those that emerge under stress).

(b) Their developmental level. Are they developmentally immature ones like emotional hunger, fear, rage, jealousy, envy, or are they developmentally more advanced ones like love, concern, empathy, anger?

(c) Their flexibility and selectivity. For example, are there many affects potentially available, some of which can selectively be called forth in the appropriate situation (fear and rage in one situation, love and empathy in another) or are there only a few (fear and rage or pseudo warmth, which are used in most situations)?

Special attention should be paid to the type of anxiety manifested:

(a) Is it related to integrated internal structural conflict, signal anxiety?

(b) Is it related to a combination of internal and external concerns (partial projection of fears onto the external world) or poorly integrated internal conflict (a fear of the instincts)?

(c) Is it related to external concerns? Fear of castration, punishment, loss of love, separation, object loss, or of annihilation by the object?

Good

There are a variety of rich, developmentally advanced affects which are selectively used in response to external or internal stimuli as well as conflict. Anxiety is related to internal integrated structural conflict (signal).

Fair
There is a capacity for advanced and selective use of affects when not under stress. Anxiety is mainly signal, but other types are experienced under extreme stress.

Marginal
A few affects predominate and are representative of pregenital concerns (emptiness, sadness, rage, envy, pseudo warmth). Anxiety is related to fear of the instincts or pregenital external concerns, separation, annihilation.

Inadequate
The affect system is not fully developed, resulting either in a lack of affect (flattening or blunting) or an inappropriateness of affect. Anxiety is related to external concerns, predominantly fear of separation, object loss, and annihilation.

4. Defenses (developmentally advanced, stable, flexible, selective, and effective vs. developmentally retarded, unstable, rigid, overly generalized and ineffective)
This category should include an assessment of the general defensive style and specific types of defenses or groups of defenses used, both ordinarily and under stress. Included should be an assessment of:

(a) Their developmental level (primitive defenses such as projection, denial, introjection vs. developmentally advanced ones such as sublimation and intellectualization)

(b) Their stability (what happens under stress)

(c) Their flexibility (how well they adapt to new situations)

(d) Their selectivity (can the most effective one be called forth for a given situation?)

(e) Their effectiveness (do they respond to signal affects, bind anxiety, and protect ego functions).

Because this is an important category which often reflects general personality functioning, a number of defenses will be listed and the rater is asked to evaluate the relative role of these or others: avoidance, withdrawal, projection, introjection, undoing, acting out, repression, identification, isolation, turning of emotions into their opposites, reaction formation, sublimation, rationalization, intellectualization, regression, and asceticism.

Good
The defenses are developmentally advanced and organized. They protect the ego without significantly hampering its functions. For

example, defenses involved in neurotic formations only minimally interfere with memory (repressed memories) or ego flexibility (repetitive reaction patterns).

Fair
The defenses are mixtures of developmentally advanced and immature defenses. Immature defenses are used mainly in response to stress. Ego functions are only compromised under stress.

Marginal
The defenses are developmentally immature (preoedipal). They hamper the ego markedly to moderately by constricting it (symptoms such as phobias, or characterological constrictions), leaving it open to severe ranges of affects (anxiety, depression), or, in cases of unusual stress, allowing disruptions in reality testing.

Inadequate
The defenses are primitive (mainly incorporation, projection, and denial), unselective, and they severely hamper basic functions (reality testing). At best they serve as only a fragile defense against psychotic processes.

* * * * * * * *

8. Relationship potential
This category should include an assessment of the individual's capacity for relationships with others. This would include an assessment of transference potential. The history of early object relationships, later relationship patterns, current patterns, and quality of affect and relatedness in the interview situation should be used as indicators.

Predominant aspects of relationship patterns should be assessed —autistic, narcissistic, anaclitic, symbiotic, sadistic, masochistic, phallic, sharing, loving, etc. Special attention should be paid to the degree to which relationships are based on pregenital dyadic patterns versus the degree to which they represent an integration of triangular oedipal patterns.

Good
Relationship patterns reflect a capacity for intimacy and stability. Pregenital traits are capable of being used in the service of genitality. There is a capacity for loving and sharing, along with capacities for assertion, self- and social boundary setting, regression, etc.

Fair
Relationships reflect some capacity for intimacy and stability, but are compromised by pregenital patterns which emerge periodically.

Marginal
There are relationships, but they are markedly unstable and are based on pregenital patterns.

REFERENCES

Bellak, L., ed. *A Concise Handbook of Community Psychiatry and Community Mental Health.* New York: Grune & Stratton, 1964.

Bruch, H. *Eating Disorders: Obesity, Anorexia Nervosa and the Person Within.* New York: Basic Books, 1973.

Greenspan, S.I. A consideration of some learning variables in the context of psychoanalytic theory: Toward a psychoanalytic learning perspective. *Psychological Issues,* IX, No. 1; Monograph #33, New York: Int. Univ. Press, January 1975.

Greenspan, S.I., and Cullander, C.C.H. A systematic metapsychological assessment of the personality—its application to the problem of analyzability. *J Am Psychoanal Assoc,* 21(2):303-327, 1973.

Mahler, M.S. *Separation-Individuation. Essays in Honor of Margaret S. Mahler.* John B. McDevitt and Calvin F. Settlage, eds., New York: Int. Univ. Press, 1971.

Mahler, M.S., and Furer, M. *On Human Symbiosis and the Viscissitudes of Individuation.* New York: Int. Univ. Press, 1968.

Piaget, J. *The Origins of Intelligence in Children.* Translated by Margaret Cook. New York: Int. Univ. Press, 1952.

CHAPTER 6

Self- and Object-Representation in Alcoholism and Other Drug-Dependence: Implications for Therapy

Henry Krystal, M.D.

For years, there was an anomaly in applying the psychoanalytic approach to addictions. On the one hand it appeared that the studies of some analysts, especially Abraham (1926), Simmel (1930, 1948) and Rado (1926, 1933), contributed insight into the psychodynamics of the drug-dependent individual. Although as analysts we continued to find evidence in psychotherapy with alcoholics that these early formulations regarding the nature of important unconscious fantasies of the patients were basically correct, the degree of success in analytic treatment of addicts was minimal. One simply could not proceed to treat the drug-dependent person in the classical psychoanalytic fashion by simply amending the list of one's interpretations with those pertaining to the oral character. The patients did not stay in treatment.

In my previous study of this problem, I came to the conclusion that there were two major areas in which drug-dependent individuals required special consideration and modification of treatment: the problems of regression in the nature of affects and affect tolerance, and certain characteristics of the drug-dependent individual self-representations and object-representations (Krystal and Raskin 1970). Elsewhere I have discussed the modifications of psychotherapy which are necessary to help the drug-dependent person to improve his affect tolerance, and start the process of affect verbalization (Krystal 1973). I consider this to be an indispensable preliminary phase of treatment for drug-dependent individuals.

This paper is concerned with the transferences, and therefore also the nature of self- and object-representations in the drug-dependent patient. First, let us look at the commonplace statement: "The object-relations of the addict are ambivalent." What is the effect of this situation on the psychotherapy? Aggression is difficult for such a patient to handle. Because of the prevalence of magical thinking, fortified by the wish for magical powers, and in harmony with a grandiose self-representation, alcoholics in psychotherapy become terrified of their death wishes directed toward the therapist. At some point in treatment they are confronted with their extraordinary envy and have the need to deal with their poorly mastered narcissistic rages. At this point, they flee from treatment, because they fear that their death wishes will destroy their therapist. Alternately, they tend to turn their aggression against themselves, and act it out in an accidental injury, suicide attempt or relapse of drinking (Simmel 1948). This may be one of the major reasons why alcoholics and drug abusers do poorly in *individual* therapy. For those alcoholics with whom individual therapy is desirable, a clinical situation works better in which auxiliary therapists are made available. As additional contacts are usually readily available in a clinic, they may be observed to be spontaneously sought by some patients with addictive problems.

The idea of using a team to manage the alcoholic patient is not new. One of the successful psychoanalytic treatment centers was Simmel's Schloss Tegel Clinic (Simmel 1948). Simmel was concerned with the alcoholic's tendency to self-punishing ideas and suicide attempts after withdrawal. The patient who was being withdrawn from alcohol was permitted to stay in bed, and a special nurse was assigned to look after him, including his diet. This was a conscious attempt to provide the patient with passive gratification, to provide a gentle "weaning" and prepare the patient for his "regular analysis" (Szasz 1958).

It has been my observation that when highly ambivalent patients have a therapeutic team available, they will use it for the purpose of "splitting" their transferences. In this way they experience their angry and destructive wishes toward one member of the team while presenting a basically loving relationship toward another, preferably the chief therapist (Krystal 1973). I believe that this happens all the time in treatment clinics and groups. However, most of the time the transferences acted out with various clinic employees will be unrecorded in a description of the therapeutic process unless a special effort is made to "gather" these. If everyone in the clinic reports to the chief therapist about *every* contact and communication with the patient, the picture of the nature of the patient's transference may then be put together. It will be found that the patient is not experiencing a simple splitting of the transference into one love and one hate relation. The picture will be quite complex, and quickly changing. At one moment, the chief therapist may be experienced as the idealized mother whose love and admiration he yearns for, while another staff member may be experienced as a rejecting, condemning parental image whom the patient dreads and hates; and still another staff member may be experienced as seductive, intrusive, destructive or other parental transference object. When the patient feels frustrated by the chief therapist, and needs to experience his rage toward him, instantly he will experience one of the other members of the team as an idealized parent, while he experiences other partial transferences with yet another clinic staff member—anybody around, whether in a therapeutic role or not. In order to demonstrate to the patient the ambivalent nature of his transference, it is necessary to bring his projections together and show that all of these transferences represent various object-representations, which he needs to experience toward the *one* therapist. The patient's vacillations and changes in attitudes toward the various staff members can be used to demonstrate his dilemma. Demonstrating the ambivalence in the transference is the crucial step in working with alcoholics, because one of the major forces which propels individuals toward addiction is that they can displace their ambivalence toward the drug. Szasz (1958) has emphasized this aspect of drug problems in his paper on the counterphobic attitude in drug dependence.

A special instance of transference splitting may occur when an alcoholic is sent to the clinic by a court. The probation officer assigned to the patient may become the object of transference of a very significant type. The fact that this type of a patient has a characterological defect, which requires that he "externalize" (that is, fail to integrate) his superego function so that others enforce controls for him, indicates that these transferences cannot be left out of the treatment (Margolis et al. 1964).

In 1931, Glover commented that drug-addicted patients are able to give up the drugs up to the very last drop. This "last drop" however, becomes virtually impossible to give up, because it contains the symbolic expression of the fantasy of taking in the love object (Glover 1931). The external object is experienced as containing the indispensable life-power which the patient wants to but cannot "internalize." This is the basic dilemma dominating the psychic reality of this type of patient. This externalizing tendency applies to his conscience as well, so that he is unable to experience it as being a part of himself but arranges for others to exercise it for him. In the use of Antabuse, we see that the fantasy solution of swallowing the object refers not only to "goodness" or narcissistic supplies, but swallowing an external source of impulse control in quite a concrete way. The failure to integrate one's own functions and aspects such as conscience, and attributing it to others, such as parents, spouses or probation officers makes the drug-dependent individual experience the world in a paranoid way. Thus, Glover remarks that drug addicts are inverted paranoids, and that they are both the persecuting and persecuted ones (1931). Whether there is a probation officer or Antabuse or similar substances (or procedures) used by the therapist, the transferences, involved in the patient's failure to see his projection of his own superego onto the external object, have to be brought into the treatment by interpretation. Otherwise the patient is never going to be able to accept himself as a whole person.

I have been talking about what I consider to be the basic defect, the basic dilemma in the life of the drug-dependent individual, such as the alcoholic. It is that he is unable to claim, own up to and exercise various parts of himself. He experiences some vital parts and functions of his own as being part of the object-representation and not self-representation. Without being consciously aware of it, he experiences himself unable to carry out these functions because he feels that this is prohibited for him, and reserved for the parental objects. I have studied and described the clinical evidence for these views elsewhere (Krystal and Raskin 1970; Krystal 1975). Let me illustrate with something that is familiar to all of us: All of us experience similarly those parts of ourselves under the control of the autonomic nervous system, which includes all of our affective expressions. We all consider these huge areas of ourselves as not being under our own control. Numerous experiments in recent years have demonstrated that through biofeedback devices one can learn to acquire conscious control of these parts. However, a surprising finding came up in our work with biofeedback combined with psychotherapy. In the psychotherapeutic relationship, we received information ordinarily lost in the biofeedback situation. Some patients experienced great anxiety over gaining control over these parts of themselves which they experienced as not meant for them. Their unconscious scheme of things was that organs such as their hearts were under the special care of God (or fate, doctor, hospital and the like) who guaranteed their survival. This is illustrated in an old-time, primitive theory of sleep—namely that God causes it by taking away the soul, which He may by His grace return to us, the next morning. This theory of sleep is a transference of the maternal image for whom lifegiving powers, as well as nursing, are reserved. This view has its roots in infancy, and even phylogeny, for certain newborn mammals will not even void unless licked by the mother (Kirk 1968). Thus, the mothering includes a permission to live by exercising certain vital functions. When the patients were told that they could be taught to control their autonomic functions, some experienced fears that taking over such maternal prerogatives would cause them to destroy themselves. Of course, even dying is viewed by some as being regulated by the mother who takes back her child (e.g., Mother Earth, or the Pieta theme) and it is a sin for one to usurp the right to end one's own life.

The reader may think I am jumping to conclusions and that biofeedback simply demonstrates a process of learning. Once the preceptive range is augmented by the apparatus, one can control extended parts of oneself. This is, of course, the learning theory as applied to biofeedback activities (DiCara 1972; Krystal 1975). But let us reexamine this premise. Experiences with hypnosis and placebo show that a subject has the potential to exercise these autonomic functions *right away* and that they are therefore not learned but are unutilized existing capacities. What happens under the influence of the hypnotist or the placebo which gives an individual the ability to exercise control over parts of himself he has hitherto reserved for his maternal transference objects?

There is a temporary lifting of internal barriers between the self-representation and the object-representation, thereby permitting access to, and control of, parts of oneself previously "walled-off." The walls curtain repressed parts of one's self, deprived of the conscious recognition of selfhood. This does not pertain just to parts of one's body but much more so to spheres of functions. Thus, just as biofeedback subjects may be reluctant to control autonomic nervous system functions even when they consciously desire it, so drug-dependents may not *want* control of appropriate self-functions.

Repressions take place at various times in childhood in connection with the various conflicts centered in psychosexual development. A boy who finds himself frightened of his competitive strivings with his father because of his fantasies and theories of destroying his father and taking his place (becoming the father) may repress these wishes and fantasies. Thereafter he may see himself as a boy, with adult masculine modes of action reserved for the father. Unless he finds some way to overcome or get around these repressions, he may never be able to fulfill his masculine ambitions, or consciously own up to, or exercise his masculinity. This would lead to the kind of inhibition in occupational and sexual goals, with a rise to prominence of homosexual striving which the early psychoanalytic writers described many times in their observations of alcoholics (Abraham 1926; Simmel 1930, 1948; Rado 1926, 1933; Juliusberger 1913; Hartmann 1925). In some homosexuals, the fantasy is that through the sexual act one will regain an alienated masculinity attributed to one's "others."

However, in drug-dependent individuals it is the "walling-off" of the maternal object-representation, and within it self-helping and comforting modes, which is the specific disturbance. Thereby, the alcoholic loses his capacity to take care of himself, to attend to his needs, to "baby" or nurse himself when tired, ill or hurt narcissistically.

In the relationship between the infant and the mother, the child gradually takes over certain functions from the mother by identification with her. Where the relationship with the mother is very troubled for the child, the maternal function becomes rigidly reserved for the mother and is experienced as prohibited for him. Some drug-dependent individuals fall into this category. But even where the relationship with the mother is good, the mother must, in addition to providing the model, communicate to the child the permission to take over these functions. An example of a type mother who has difficulty in permitting this can be observed in the nursery where some mothers become "jealous" of the child's transitional object, and punish the child or prevent its use for self-comforting. Those things which the child does to comfort himself, from thumbsucking to masturbation, each provide an occasion for communication of the permissibility of utilizing self-comforting modes of behavior. When a person feels that he cannot (actually may not) exercise these functions, he feels envious of his mother, and other women, and transference objects, e.g., doctors, and yearns to gain them symbolically or magically.

Therein is the source of the drive by the alcoholic to use the drug, both as a pharmacological means to manipulate his affective states and as a placebo, to gain surcease from his feelings of depletion resulting from the repression[1] of self-helping attributes and functions of his own by making it part of a rigidly walled-off object-representation. We must recognize and acknowledge that the kind of person who is likely to become drug dependent is one who uses the drug to help him carry out basic survival functions which

---

[1] I have discussed elsewhere the concept of repression as referred to in this context. It extends the definition of elements repressed from those rendered unconscious, to include those alienated: not consciously recognizable as part of one's self and one's own living (Krystal 1973).

he otherwise cannot do. People who drink in order to be able to continue to work, thus gain access to their assertive, masculine, paternal modes of behavior. People who drink for the purpose of surcease and comfort obtain their goal, in addition to the pharmacological effects, by gaining access and ability to exercise their maternal functions. The longing to regain alienated parts of oneself is the real meaning behind the fantasies of fusion with the good mother so clearly discernible in drug-dependent individuals (Chessick 1960; Savitt 1963).

These yearnings make their appearance in the transference in psychotherapy with alcoholics and other drug-dependent individuals, and in this phase of the treatment, the phenomenon has been termed by Fenichel "object addiction" (1945). This transference needs to be interpreted in psychotherapy for the same reason that all transferences need to be interpreted: So that the patient will discover that the characteristics which he attributes to the analyst (psychotherapist) are actually his own mental representations which he first perceived as being part of his mother, and now reexperiences again, attributing them to the therapist. The healing principle of psychoanalysis consists in the patients claiming their own mind, restoring the inviolable unity of their own selves.

But, as we know too well, patients do not feel free to do this. They fight it with all the means at their disposal, as if their lives depended on maintaining the repressions. And of all patients, drug-dependent individuals have the worst struggle with this part of treatment. When we try to understand the nature of their psychic reality, which made the removal of repression of their maternal object-representations so difficult for them, we discover that it leads to care of their emotional problems derived from infantile traumata.

However, first let us step back and take another look at one aspect of drug addiction so obvious that we take it for granted, and thereby miss an essential clue to the nature of the intrapsychic conflict in alcoholism as well as other related states. Drug abuse consists in fact, not only of taking drugs, but equally important, being deprived of drug effect. Drugs which are addicting are short acting. The longer acting the drug, the greater the likelihood of the user panicking and developing a "bum trip" (Krystal and Raskin 1970).

Withdrawal from drugs is an integral part of the process of addiction (Krystal 1962). The development of ever-increasing tolerance for the drug is greater and faster in drug-dependent individuals because they have the need to deprive the drug of its power (Krystal 1966), at the same time, the moment it does lose its force, they panic (Rado 1933; Krystal 1962).

What is the meaning of all of these apparent contradictions? It is that *while the drug-dependent yearns for the union with his maternal love object (representation), he also dreads it.* He really can't stand it either way. Schizophrenic patients and some borderline individuals yearn for union with their love object (representation) and once they achieve it (in fantasy), they cling to it passionately, giving up conscious registration of all contacts with whatever might spoil it.

Drug-dependent individuals are very busy getting the drug, but can feel themselves reunited with the idealized love object only rarely for short periods of time, and only at moments when they are virtually totally anesthetized. And even then, one finds with amazement that many of them—at the very moment of the climactic action of the drug—indulge in acts of riddance, such as moving bowels, vomiting, cleaning their bodies, cutting their nails, or even house cleaning (Chessick 1960). It may be said that they are *addicted to the process of taking in and losing the drug rather than to having* it. The seemingly bizarre behavior of the drug addict who plays with the drug by "regurgitating" it back and forth between the syringe and vein suddenly falls into place here.

Drug-dependent individuals dread fusion with the love object representations because of the way they experienced them in the formative period of their lives. Their mothering was unsatisfactory, with resulting severe psychic traumatization in infancy, and many and wide-ranging damaging effects to their personalities. As a result, whatever one looks for, one finds.

When the early analysts were fascinated by their discovery of the psychosexual development, they found that alcoholics were fixated on the oral level (Abraham 1954). When they paid attention to the nature of unconscious fantasies, they discovered yearning for union, as well as persecutory fears (Simmel 1948; Rado 1926; Szasz 1958). When they became aware of the role of homosexual striving in the genesis of emotional problems, alcoholics were found to have them and dread them (Hartmann 1925). When they became aware of characterology, alcoholics were found to be schizoid characters (Simmel 1930), in addition to the earlier classification of them as oral characters. When they started paying attention to ego functions, these were found to be impaired as well (Savitt 1963).

I have made two additions to this wealth of views of the nature of psychological disturbances of drug-dependent individuals:

(1) I have found that as a result of massive childhood psychic trauma, these individuals experienced arrest in affect development and an impairment of affect tolerance (Krystal 1970, 1974, 1975). These produce, in effect, a fear of feelings, and need to block them.

(2) I found that in order to survive, some drug-dependent individuals had to repress their rage and destructive wishes toward their maternal love object. This manifests itself in a rigid "walling-off" of the maternal love object representation, especially with an idealization of it, and an attribution of most of life-supporting and nurturing functions to it. By doing this, the patient manages (in his fantasy) to protect the love object from his fantasied destructive powers, and assure that "someone *out there*" loved him and would take care of him (Krystal and Raskin 1970).

But the repressed aggression never disappears, and so the alcoholic and other drug addicts dread that if they accomplish fusion with the love object they will destroy it, and thereby return themselves to a traumatic situation, which they dread. One clinical observation well known to every worker in this field supports the accuracy of these constructions: Patients are unable to accomplish normally the work of mourning and the feeling of "introjecting" the lost love object. The introjection fantasy is a form of partial union of the self-representation and object-representation, which most people achieve at the end of mourning. It is a clinical commonplace to say that alcoholics and other drug-dependent individuals cannot tolerate object losses (and that includes therapists) without being so threatened with their own affects that they have a virtually unavoidable relapse to self-destructive drug use.

This is the dimension of the problem of ambivalence which makes its appearance in psychotherapy with alcoholics. In the early stages of therapy the very availability of an object creates serious challenges to the patient. There is the already mentioned fear of aggressive impulses and wishes. There is, in addition, the problem stressed by Vaillant (1974), that when alcoholic patients idealize their therapists in the transference, they experience themselves as worthless and bad.

But these are just preliminaries. The greatest difficulty is that effective work in (intensive, psychoanalytically oriented) psychotherapy, through which one can give up attachment to infantile object-representations and the infantile view of oneself, is by "effective grieving," a process analogous to mourning (Wetmore 1963). That very process spells trouble for the drug-dependent patient, who tends to dread being overwhelmed with depression, which represents to him the return to childhood trauma. Raskin and I postulate, in order to explain this phenomenon, that this type of individual has had a nearly destructive childhood trauma experience, which he fears may return, and which he experiences as a "fate worse than death" (Krystal and Raskin 1970). Elsewhere I have discussed the *technical* modifications made necessary by regression in the nature of affects and impairment of affect tolerance. If even that obstacle is overcome, and the patient is able to grieve effectively, then he faces the ultimate challenge: the conscious acceptance of his object-representations as his own mental creations. At the end of a successful analysis one is in the same position as at the end of the hypothetical completely successful mourning. The bereaved person discovers that though the lost person is dead and gone, he continues to exist in the survivor's mind. This gives him the opportunity to discover that as far as he is concerned, that is where the object had been all along—in his mind as an object-representation of his own creation. And so one has to face the "return of the repressed." All the "bad" persecutory aspects of the object could be viewed as projections, but they are really simply fantasies, impulses, wishes and feelings which were not integrated. In other words, the giving up of the repressions, the owning up to the self-sameness of one's object-representations confronts one with the aggression which caused the alcoholic to "wall-off" his object-representation so rigidly, and subsequently to develop that tragic yearning and dread of the love object.

Earlier I said that the rigid "walling-off" of the maternal object-representation took place in the face of extreme aggressive impulses toward it. The evidence for that came from this stage of the psycho-therapeutic work with drug-dependent individuals. The intensity of the narcissistic rages, the persistence of the aggressive impulses make one wonder if all addiction is, at bottom a "hate-addiction." The problem of aggression and its apparent threat to the safety and integrity of the self-representation and/or object-representation sets the limits to the kinds and numbers of drug-dependent patients who can be carried to completion of psychotherapy. Along the way most such patients, when confronted with their aggression, will relapse again and again into drug use and self-destructive activities. Others will be driven to prove that their childhood misfortunes were *real*, by getting the therapist angry and provoking abuse. Still others become so terrified of the dangerous, poisonous transference object, that they set out on a panicked, frantic search for the *ideal mother* in some form—such as drink, love or gambling. If the therapist is otherwise equipped to bear the disappointments, provocations and failures entailed in working with these patients, and has the time and patience to permit the patient to do this work by minute steps, then it is helpful to keep in mind that the patient is confronted with problems of aggression that make him experience the transference as a life-and-death struggle. Care and caution must be exercised that the patient not be overwhelmed with his aggressive feelings, or guilt. Emergencies in which the patient's life hangs in the balance will occur, for that may be the way the patient may have to test the therapist.

When Simmel reviewed his lifetime experience with alcoholics in a paper which he never completed, he was very clear about the problems of aggression in the treatment of these patients. He said:

> ... during a state of abstinence under psychoanalysis in a hospital, substituting for the addiction to alcohol or drugs was an overt suicidal addiction or an overt addiction to homicide. During this stage the addict's only compulsion is to kill: himself or others. Usually he does not rationalize this urge; he just wants to die or, at other times he just wants to kill (Simmel 1948, p. 24).

The aggression observable in the self-destructive lifestyle of the drug-dependent individual is, in the process of psychotherapy, traced to its ultimate sources and meanings. In this process the patient has to be able to experience with the therapist that which he has never dared to face—his hatred. Instead of seeing himself as a victim, and claiming *innocence*, now he confronts his murderous aggression. To do so, however, requires giving up the treasured view of oneself as the innocent victim, which again, has to be mourned. And so, it can be said that an unavoidable step in the treatment of a certain type of drug-dependent individual in intensive therapy is a depressive stage. During this phase of the treatment the dependence upon the therapist is extreme, and no substitutes are acceptable. While early in the treatment many patients do best in a clinic with multiple therapists, for the few who will be carried to this type of therapeutic completion, the chief therapist has to be the one who will be stationary and available to the very end.

Such are some of the difficulties resulting from the nature of object-representation in addictive personalities. They determine that successful psychoanalytic psychotherapy will continue to be the exception, mainly of research interest.

SUMMARY

The nature of the object relations of the drug-dependent patient is such that he craves to be united with ideal object, but at the same time dreads it. He thus becomes addicted to acting out the drama of fantasy introjection and separation from the drug. There is a corresponding intrapsychic defect; certain essential functions related to nurturance are reserved for the object-representation. The objective of therapy is to permit the patient to extend his conscious self-recognition to all of himself, thereby freeing him from the need for the placebo effect of the drug as a means of gaining access to his alienated parts and functions.

REFERENCES

Abraham, K. The influence of oral erotism on character formation. In: *Selected Papers of Karl Abraham*. New York: Basic Books, 1954.

_____. The psychological relation between sexuality and alcoholism. *Int J Psychoanal*, 7:2, 1926.

Chessick, R.D. The pharmacogenic orgasm. *Arch Gen Psychiatry*, 3:117-128, 1960.

Clark, L.P. Psychological study of some alcoholics. *Psychoanal Rev*, 6:268, 1919.

DiCara, L. Learning mechanisms. In: *Biofeedback and Self-Control*. Chicago: Aldine, 1972.

Fenichel, O. *The Psychoanalytic Theory of the Neuroses*. New York: Norton, 1945.

Glover, E. The prevention and treatment of drug addiction. *Br J of Inebriety*, 29:13-18, 1931.

Hartmann, H. Cocainismus und homosexualitat. *Z Neur*, 95:415, 1925.

Juliusberger, O. Psychology of alcoholism. *Zentralblatt fur psychoanal*, 3:1, 1913. Abstract in *Psychoanal Rev*, 1:469, 1913-14.

Kirk, R.W. Pediatrics. In: *Canine Medicine*, Earl J. Catcott, ed. Santa Barbara, CA: Amer. Vet. Pub., Inc., 1968, p. 809.

Krystal, H. The physiological basis of the treatment of delirium tremens. *Am J Psychiatry*, 116:137-147, 1959.

_____. The study of withdrawal from narcotics as a state of stress. *Psychoanal Q Suppl*, 36:53-65, 1962.

_____. Therapeutic assistants in psychotherapy with regressed patients. In: *Current Psychiatric Therapies*, J. Masserman, ed., 1964, p. 232.

_____. Withdrawal from drugs. *Psychosomatics*, 7:199-302, 1966.

_____. Technical Modification in Affect Regression and Impairment of Affect Tolerance. Paper presented at the Annual Meeting of the American Psychoanalytic Association, 1973.

_____. Psychic Reality. Paper presented to the Michigan Psychoanalytic Society on March 1, 1973. Mimeographed.

_____. The genetic development of affects and affect regression. Part I. *The Annual of Psychoanalysis*, Vol. II, 1974.

_____. The genetic development of affects and affect regression. Part II. Affect tolerance. *The Annual of Psychoanalysis*, Vol. III., p. 179-219, 1975.

Krystal, H. and Raskin, H.A. *Drug Dependence: Aspects of Ego Function*. Detroit: Wayne State Univ Press, 1970.

Margolis, M., Krystal, H., and Siegel, S. Psychotherapy with alcoholic offenders. *Q J Alcoh*, 25:85-99, 1964.

Rado, S. The psychic effect of intoxicants: An attempt to evolve a psychoanalytic theory of morbid craving. *Int J Psychoanal*, 7:396-413, 1926. (Also in: *Psychoanalysis of Behavior*. New York: Grune & Stratton, 1956.)

_____. The psychoanalysis of pharmacothymia. *Psychoanal Q*, 2:1-3, 1933. (Also in *Psychoanalysis of Behavior*.)

Savitt, R.A. Psychoanalytic studies on addiction: Ego structure in narcotic addicts. *Psychoanal Q*, 32:43-57, 1963.

Simmel, E. Morbid habits and cravings. *Psychoanal Rev*, 17:48-54, 1930.

_____. Alcoholism and addiction. *Psychoanal Q*, 17:6-31, 1948.

Stoyva, J. The public (scientific) study of private events. In: *Biofeedback and Self-Control*, Barber, T.X., ed. Chicago: Aldine, 1970.

Szasz, T.S. The counterphobic mechanisms in addiction. *J Am Psychoanal Assoc*, 6:309-325, 1958.

Vaillant, G. Paper on The Treatment of Alcoholics in the Cambridge Alcoholic Clinic. Given at a Symposium on Alcoholism, Boston Univ, 1974.

Wetmore, R.J. The role of grief in psychoanalysis. *Int J Psychoanal*, 44:97-103, 1963.

CHAPTER 7

The Ego, the Self, and Opiate Addiction: Theoretical and Treatment Considerations

Edward J. Khantzian, M.D.

INTRODUCTION

Until recently, the psychoanalytic literature on addiction stressed the pleasurable aspects of drug use to explain the compelling nature of addiction (Abraham 1960; Freud 1955; Rado 1933, 1957). Although Rado and others (Fenichel 1945; Savitt 1954; Wikler and Rasor 1953) appreciated underlying factors of depression, tension, and anxiety, many of these same workers continued to place particular emphasis on the euphoric-pleasurable aspects of drug use. Most of this literature on addiction focuses on the regressive gratification of libidinal instincts achieved through the use of addictive substances. Glover's work stands in striking contrast to the other theoretical explanations of addiction. He stressed that addicts used their substance progressively (as opposed to regressively) to defend against primitive, sadistic impulses and to avoid psychosis. He seemed to appreciate better the enormous difficulties addicts have with their aggression and viewed the sexual and pleasurable aspects of drug use as defensive responses to the underlying problems with aggression (Glover 1956).

More recent works (Chein et al. 1964; Khantzian 1974a, 1974b, 1975; Krystal and Raskin 1970; Milkman and Frosch 1973; Wieder and Kaplan 1969; Wurmser 1974) have stressed the adaptive use of drugs and have tried to incorporate a better appreciation of how the psychopharmacologic action of the different drugs interacts with the personality organization of addicted individuals. These reports have focused on ego functions and ego impairments, and in particu-

101

lar on problems which affect tolerance (Krystal and Raskin 1970; Wurmser 1974) and drive defense (Khantzian 1974a). Zinberg (1975) has stressed the importance of setting and how it interacts with ego function and drug effect. Some of these reports have also tried to take into account narcissistic problems that contribute to the individual's general predisposition to addiction, and to some of the related specific ego impairments and psychopathology that are evident in addicted individuals.

In this report I will selectively review and expand on recent theoretical and clinical investigative work that has focused on the ego impairments of narcotic addicts, particularly in relation to problems of affect and drive defense. I will also attempt to explore how certain problems with self-care and self-regulation are related to failures in internalization, and how these failures in development leave such individuals vulnerable to a whole range of hazardous behavior and involvements, but in particular to addictions. Finally, an attempt will be made to examine certain unique and characteristic traits which are related to narcissistic processes and defense so common among addicts. These characteristics serve to compensate for their developmental impairments, but at the same time impede such individuals in establishing and obtaining sufficient satisfactions in their involvement with people, work and play. On the basis of these theoretical considerations, some implications for treatment interventions will be explored.

AFFECT AND DRIVE DEFENSE

In working with narcotic addicts one often hears the claim that they are psychologically "healthier" than other types of addicts or psychiatric patients. Such claims are bolstered by arguments that one would have to be healthier and "better put together" to survive the challenges and dangers involved in obtaining the money and drugs to support an addiction to heroin. Such claims are based on observations of how successful such individuals seem to be in acting upon and extracting from their surroundings what they want for themselves. This apparent "success" distracts both the observer and the addict from indications of failure in functioning that are often equally as apparent, namely, the addict's inability to cope with his emotions and his relations with other people. The so-called "successful" functioning of the heroin addict says less about his/her mental health than about how the ego of such individuals is shaped and developed along certain lines to serve their addiction and related requirements. However, we also suspect that these special qualities of addicts represent attempts to make up for and to offset major deficits, impairments and failures in defense against their affects and drives.

We believe these failures and deficits in defense are developmental and are intimately related to problems with internalization. Internalization is a process by which the developing infant and child acquires qualities and functions from parental figures in the process of maturation. Ideally, the person eventually can care for himself as a result of this internalization. This process is probably related to the ways in which the developing person is exposed to the "good enough (caring) environment" and how "the good enough mothering" in infancy and childhood gets into the person as a function of adequate nurturing (Winnicott 1953). If successful, this process of internalization establishes within the person a coherent sense of the self, an appreciation of the separate existence of others, as well as the establishment of adequate ego functions that serve purposes of defense and adaption. In this section, I will focus on those aspects of internalization related to ego mechanisms of defense, especially against affects and drives, and we will stress particularly ego impairments and problems associated with drive and affect defense in narcotic addicts.

Based on direct child observation, and clinical practice with adults, there is rather convincing evidence that normal development requires certain amounts of frustration (Kohut 1971; Mahler 1968; Meissner, Mack, and Semrad 1975; Winnicott 1953). Optimally, extremes of deprivation or indulgence are avoided and the child is confronted with enough tolerable disappointment that a capacity to tolerate emotional distress and pain is gradually built up. To summarize how this capacity evolves, the individual gradually incorporates into a sense of the self and into the ego the parents' protective role and their function as a stimulus barrier. Used in this sense, "stimulus barrier" refers to those aspects of ego functions that operate either to maintain a minimal level of unpleasant affects or tension, or to defend against such feelings through appropriate action and mechanisms of defense when they reach high or intolerable levels.

Krystal and Raskin (1970) have traced how affects also develop along certain lines and serve the ego to defend against internal emotional states and drives. They have delineated in a most helpful way how anxiety and depression develop out of a common undifferentiated matrix, and evolve through differentiation, desomatization and verbalization. Ideally, this process of development ultimately allows the person to use feelings as a guide and signal to mobilize the ego in response to the constant barrage of internal and external stimuli involved in human living. They further review how trauma in the course of development (or as a result of catastrophic events later in life) may lead to both affective disturbances and drug dependence. They stress how traumatization produces a reversal and regression resulting in de-differentiation of affects. In addition to trauma, they also stress how the failure of parents to act as adequate models in managing affects leads to an arrest in development, which precludes successful differentiation. In the case of addicts, a major consequence of such development arrest is that they are unable to make use of anxiety and feelings as signals or guides because their feelings are undifferentiated and overwhelming.

Krystal and Raskin are fully aware of the specific anesthetic action of heroin on painful affects and explain most cogently why individuals involved with heroin are subject to and are unable to manage overwhelming affect states. However, in my estimation, they do not sufficiently distinguish the action of opiates from other sedatives and alcohol. In addition to its antiaggression action, I believe that the capacity of heroin, specifically, to relieve overwhelming, distressful affect states is what makes it such a compelling substance for narcotic addicts. This observation might seem to state the obvious, but to specify and more precisely define what affect states are relieved by heroin and other drugs has most important implications for management and treatment, especially with psychotropic drugs.

Kohut (1971) has traced how problems with internalization are linked to narcissistic disturbances, and in particular, how such disturbances lie at the root of addictive disorders. A child's traumatic disappointments with the mother because of her lack of empathy, her failure to act as an adequate stimulus barrier or to provide adequate stimuli and gratification of tension, lead to a failure in development of the child's psychic apparatus. Later in life many of these individuals discover that drugs substitute for defects in their ability to cope with inevitable life distresses and disappointments. Kohut makes the provocative statement, *"the drug—serves not as a substitute for loved or loving objects, or for a relationship with them, but as a replacement for a defect in the psychological structure"* (p. 46) (emphasis added). Wieder and Kaplan (1969) similarly appreciate this aspect of drug use referring to drugs as a "corrective—and prosthetic." Wurmser (1974) comes to the same conclusion, referring to the addict's "defect of affect defense." He emphasizes the addict's enormous difficulties in handling painful affects, and how opiates in particular act to relieve feelings of narcissistic rage, shame, hurt, and loneliness. In lieu of adequate defenses, Wurmser speculates that narcotics act by damping such feelings directly and/ or raising the threshold against reactions of narcissistic disappointment.

A recent case example highlights nicely some of the problems with internalization and defects in affect defense that have been reviewed thus far:

A 29-year-old male was struggling with much rage and anxiety. Despite all good intentions, he found himself reverting to previous addictive behavior. His reversion had occurred in the context of a visit from his mother, whom he had not seen in over a year. She had reprimanded him about some recent financial indiscretions that concerned her, but had totally failed to appreciate how anxious, fragmented, and overwhelmed he was feeling at the time. The painful consequences of the defects in his ego structure and the quality of the overwhelming feelings in the absence of such structure were poignantly conveyed in the account of his reactions to his mother's visit. He also gave some hints about how such deficits originate in parental attitudes and disappointment. He complained—"My mother is utterly disregarding. She doesn't know me at all—what I feel or think or what I'm like. When I feel anxious, I feel it all over, not just butterflies in my stomach or sweaty hands. I feel it all over. When I get anxious, I get anxiouser, and anxiouser and anxiouser. When I get afraid, the only thing that makes it go away—" and then he struggled to explain, and finally offered—"is a stronger person." In this context he pleaded that the therapist prescribe a medication for his anxiety.

In my own work with narcotic addicts, I have been impressed with the lifelong difficulties such individuals have had with aggression and derivative problems with rage and depression. After obtaining repeated histories from addicts about how dysphoric feelings associated with restlessness, anger and rage were relieved by heroin and other opiates, and after observing narcotic addicts stabilize on methadone, I began to suspect that narcotics might have a direct antiaggression action. In a previous report (Khantzian 1974a) I summarized these findings and concluded that problems with aggression predisposed certain individuals to dependence on opiates and played a central role in the development of addiction. I stressed the addict's use of the antiaggression action of opiates in the service of drive defense, and formulated how the longer but same action of methadone was the basis for "success" of methadone maintenance. In the report cited and elsewhere (Khantzian 1972), we stressed the disorganizing influence of aggression on ego function in individuals whose ego stability was already subject to dysfunction and impairment either as a result of developmental arrest or regression.[1]

Although our own work with narcotic addicts has stressed problems with drive defense, particularly in relation to aggressive drives, it is important to note and emphasize that all the more recently cited reports of clinical investigative work with narcotic addicts are remarkably consistent with each other. They stress problems with drive and affect defense and focus on developmental impairments in the ego. More remarkable, much of this consensus has been arrived at almost simultaneously and independently. I believe that further work on the "ego side" of the problem, with cross fertilization of thinking among various investigators promises to yield further understanding of the relationship between drive and affect states, and various ego defenses and modes of adaptation. Milkman and Frosch (1973), for example, have recently reported on a promising line of inquiry in applying to addicts a systematic study of ego functions developed by Bellak and Hurvich. Their preliminary findings show a relationship between an abuser's characteristic mode of adaptation and his/her preference for either amphetamines or heroin.

We have said little up to this point specifically about character pathology, and yet we know that our patients most often are referred to as "psychopaths, sociopaths, and antisocial characters." I believe these labels, so often used pejoratively, describe little that is meaningful or accurate about addicts. Perhaps such descriptions mostly indicate how little we understand character pathology. I suspect that as we study such problems, we will gain a better appreciation of the relationship between various drive and affect states and the ways in which such states contribute to or "drive" so-called character pathology and related behavioral disorder such as narcotic addiction. In my work with character problems, I am in agreement with the proposition offered by Vaillant (1975) and Wishnie (1974), that as control is gained over the behavior problems, underlying psychopathology that was previously masked by the destructive behavior emerges. Vaillant and Wishnie stress in particular the underlying depression. My own experience not only emphasizes the

---

[1]Zinberg has questioned seriously the role of preexisting psychopathology as a major determinant of addiction. He has perceptively and persuasively proposed that regression in addicts is less a function of personality disturbance and drug effect, but more, the result of being labeled as deviant, the loss of varied contact with social and family relationships and the necessity to "cop." Although his work is at variance with the emphasis on developmental impairments in this report, his point of view is not incompatible with what we have proposed. His study reminds us of the importance of "stimulus nutriment" from the environment in maintaining autonomous ego functions (Zinberg 1975).

underlying depression, but the presence as well of a range and variety of mood disorders, phobic-anxious states and other neurotic, characterologic, and psychotic symptoms. As we more precisely identify such target symptoms and affect states, we will be in a better position to decide on suitable forms and types of psychological and psychopharmacologic interventions.

SELF-CARE AND SELF-REGULATION[2]

In this section I would like to explore in a preliminary way an aspect of addiction which seems to have received little systematic attention in the literature, related to a particular type of gap or vulnerability in ego function of drug-dependent individuals. Namely, I have been impressed with an apparent disregard that drug-dependent individuals show for a whole range of real or possible dangers to their well-being, including their substance involvement. I believe this type of self-disregard is associated with impairments of a generic or global ego function that I have chose to designate as *self-care and self-regulation*. I say "generic or global" because I suspect such functions and their impairments are related to component ego functions such as signal anxiety, reality testing, judgment, control, and synthesis, and when impaired, to such defenses as denial, justification, projection, etc. As used here, the concept of self-care combines elements of all of these component functions and in this respect it is a complex function. But in other respects the functions of self-care and regulation are so basic and elementary for survival that they are sufficiently developed and present to be evident in normal young children.

Before proceeding to elaborate on problems of self-care as an ego function, I would like to stress what I am *not* referring to or emphasizing in this discussion. Considerable references exist in the literature to the obvious self-destructive nature of addictions. Often in such cases reference is made to unconscious "death wishes." In other cases, referred to in the previous section, the apparent disregard and "not caring" is related to desperate attempts to ward off painful feelings. In still other instances dangerous and violent behavior serves to counteract feelings of helplessness and dependency, and as Wieder and Kaplan have correctly indicated, it is a mode that is adopted against one's sense of terror and vulnerability. In these cases the actual and potential problems and danger for the person

---

[2]The author is indebted to Dr. John E. Mack for his assistance in the development of the germinal idea and concept of self-care as an ego function.

are driven, over-determined, and defensive. These self-destructive aspects of addiction have received considerable attention and will not be the main focus of our attention.

For purposes here, I will stress how much of the addict's self-disregard is not so much consciously or unconsciously motivated, but more a reflection of defects in self-care functions as a result of failures to adopt and internalize these functions from the caring parents in early and subsequent phases of development. The over-determined and defensive forms of self-destructive behavior among addicts do not adequately account for all the terribly dangerous and destructive activity, to the point of death, that such people get into. In such cases danger is not so much consciously or unconsciously welcomed, or counterphobically denied, but rather is never anticipated, perceived and/or appreciated. These are problems that I consider to be related to self-care (ego) functions that are impaired, deficient and/or absent in so many of the addicts we see. The problems with self-care and regulation are apparent in their past histories (pre-dating their addiction) by a high incidence of preventable medical and dental problems, accidents, fights and violent behavior, and delinquent/behavioral problems. Their impaired self-care function is also evident in relation to their drug problems, where despite obvious deterioration and imminent danger as a result of their drug use, there is little evidence of fear, anxiety or realistic assessment about their substance involvement. One might correctly argue that in this latter instance the lack of self-care is secondary to regression as a result of prolonged drug use. Although this is probably quite true, we have been impressed with the presence and persistence of these described tendencies in such individuals both prior to becoming addicted, and subsequent to becoming drug free and stabilized. In fact much of our therapeutic work beyond detoxification involves the work of helping our patients to identify these impairments around self-care, and to help them learn to incorporate these functions for the first time in their daily living and behavior.

In contrast to the compulsive aspects of drug use where drugs come into a person's life to serve purposes of defense and adaptation, some of the more malignant aspects of drug addiction that we are stressing here are related to the impulsive, maladaptive side of the problem. That is, the addiction to drugs and the associated involvements and activities, that are often equally as dangerous, represent a failure in the person's ego to properly assess, warn, and protect the individual against the dangers in a whole variety of settings and situations, not the least of which is the setting associated with addictions.

Some examples taken from a women's correctional institution where most of the individuals have been drug free and relatively stable for some time are presented for purposes of illustration.[3]

Some of the most telling examples are evident in relation to health issues: failure to clean needles that are shared is common; gross dietary indiscretions such as the diabetic failing to adhere to a proper diet or an inmate's buying the most spicy foods despite a chronic ulcer; failures in the sexual sphere to take precautions against pregnancy or to worry about the possibility of venereal disease, or to obtain regular gynecologic examinations.

Then there are people who "just happen to be in the wrong place at the wrong time." For example, one inmate went shopping with her boyfriend and was arrested for shoplifting after the boyfriend asked her to hold a bag containing a suit he had shoplifted. Another woman landed in jail because she believed her male friend, who told her that she was just "live parking" the car while he went to the bank, when in fact she was driving the getaway car.

Another inmate went for a walk with a girlfriend whom she knew was planning to shoplift. She was caught and arrested for shoplifting and protested that she was "only going along for the fresh air" and couldn't figure out why she was charged.

In our own drug program we have been impressed with the many 11th hour lapses, oversights, mistakes and crises in which patients find themselves, that undermine employment opportunities and treatment and education plans that the patient and the program staff have worked hard to realize.

In all of the examples it is not uncommon to hear such people reply, "I didn't think about it," when questioned as to how they could leave themselves so vulnerable. Usually, our dynamic formulations about such behavior stress such consideration as regression, unconscious wishes, conflict, denial and repetition compulsion. I believe these formulations do a disservice to understanding the problems of these individuals. These explanations fail to consider at face value that the apparent oblivion in their "not thinking" statements accurately reflects the locus of the problem. To quote from

---

[3]The author is indebted to Dr. Catherine Treece for these vignettes and case examples.

another report, we summarized the problem as follows: "Although much of this behavior is dynamically motivated and defensive in nature, as well as symptomatic of regression, in other respect these individuals' apparent self-disregard ("thoughtlessness"), delinquency, failure to comply with assigned treatment plans, missed appointments, tardiness, etc., reflect a particular kind of absence and impairment in ego function, that predisposes people to mishaps and mistakes. These are functions which when better established, either automatically guide most of us away from trouble, or once in trouble, these and similar ego functions are mobilized, again fairly automatically, to direct us out of trouble" (Khantzian and Kates 1976).

In my opinion, it is specifically around this kind of impairment that we need to structure treatment programs. We must provide measures that actively and directly both respond to the overdetermined need to fend off help, and deal with the tendency of these individuals to be insufficiently anxious, concerned, and responsive about so many aspects of their life, but especially, about self-care measures.

As indicated previously, our description of self-care and regulation as an ego function probably consists of elements, components, and processes related to other ego functions. In our estimation the adoption of a construct such as self-care as a possible unique ego function has particular utility and explanatory value in trying to understand behavioral problems in general and the maladaptive aspects of addiction in particular. This function is related to signal anxiety, and along lines developed by Krystal and Raskin (1970), serves to guide us in relation to external dangers, threats and involvements. Krystal and Raskin stress the role of signal anxiety in relation to internal states and how in its absence the individual tends to be overcome by overwhelming affects. With self-care functions, our emphasis is on the person's external world and his surroundings; when self-care functions are inadequate, the individual fails to perceive or judge realistically various dangers and threats. This function and its impairments are also related to ego functions involving "synthesis" and bear many similarities to this function as explained and applied by Chein et al. (1964) to the ego impairment of narcotic addicts. However, we believe this emphasis on self-care as an ego function, with the emphasis on external dangers and threats, is warranted because both the concepts of signal anxiety and synthetic functions stress intrapsychic processes and mechanisms, and fail to stress sufficiently and take into account the individual's adaptation to reality and the world around him.

THE SELF AND NARCISSISTIC DEFENSE

In this section I would like to focus briefly on some distinctive character features and traits common among addicts. In the previous two sections of this paper we have stressed ego mechanisms that serve a *function* in personality organization and adaptation. In this section, *attitudes* about the self and others, and the ways in which such attitudes are incorporated into character traits/styles will be stressed. Kohut (1971) and Kernberg (1975) have recently elaborated on how disturbances in early child rearing, especially around nurturance and dependency needs, lead to narcissistic disturbances in adult life. (Narcissism refers to new scientific work on the self, including the vicissitudes of its development and its ultimate deficiencies or intactness—ed.) Although both Kohut and Kernberg have indicated that narcissistic pathology predisposes certain individuals to addiction, neither has systematically explored the relationship between narcissistic disturbances and addiction. Wurmser has made a major contribution by expanding on this work and carefully reviewing the narcissistic basis for defects in affect defense, faulty ego ideal formation, pathological dependency and enormous problems that addicts have with rage, shame, hurt and loneliness.

Wurmser's work (1974) has placed emphasis on narcissistic decompensation and the part that drugs play in allaying and countering painful affect states and narcissistic disturbances that result from an overwhelming crisis in the individual's life. In my own work, I have recently become interested in trying to identify and understand better some of the unique and characteristic traits of *compensated* addicts that are related to narcissistic processes and disturbances. More specifically, in psychotherapeutic work with stabilized addicts (i.e., post-detoxified or on drug maintenance) I have been interested in exploring some of the special qualities and problems addicts display in obtaining satisfactions of their needs. Despite their totally and/or relatively drug-free state, extreme and often alternating patterns of reactions in relation to their need satisfactions persist. In the therapeutic relationship, the most commonly observed feature is the extent to which such patients go to be compliant, cooperative, and most of all, what little demand the patient places on the therapist for very long periods of time. Most often this takes such forms as passivity, indifference, solicitousness, disavowal, and self-sufficiency.

Occasionally, such patients lapse and display another side to themselves, for example, a most inappropriate intrusiveness into the life and activities of the therapist, and an assumption that their curiosity will or ought to be satisfied; on other occasions a request will be made that superficially sounds innocent and undemanding, but actually reveals an enormous sense of entitlement and total lack of appreciation about the magnitude and sensitivity of their request. One such patient in the course of his employment discovered he needed some confidential information on a person who was affiliated with an institution in which the therapist worked. In a matter-of-fact way he asked the therapist to obtain this information for him. He seemed totally surprised and hurt when he was tactfully informed that his request was unreasonable.

Most of these same patterns carry over to their everyday life. In reviewing these patterns with such patients one discovers that many of their complaints of boredom, depression and dissatisfaction are related to these same rigidly maintained patterns of self-denial observable in their small demands in therapy. At other times one hears accounts of massive explosions of anger and frustration as a result of chancing some wish or want and then experiencing massive disappointment.

Kernberg (1975) has stressed mechanisms of splitting and primitive dissociation in narcissistic disturbances, where for example, seemingly opposite ego attitudes of shyness and arrogance may coexist. Kohut has emphasized massive repression and disavowal of needs to describe how narcissistic personalities attempt to defend against their passive wishes and wants. These are not at all uncommon characteristics and modes of defense in narcotic addicts with whom I have worked; and I believe these characteristics account for so much of the unevenness in function, and unpredictability and contradiction in attitudes in such patients. In one patient the following characteristics have been persistently and simultaneously evident:

Solicitous—When he first came for treatment, he went out of his way to be extremely chatty and friendly with all the secretaries in a nearby administrative area. He has always gone out of his way to light people's cigarettes, including that of his therapist. When the therapist has been late, he has never complained, and more often goes out of his way to dismiss any resulting inconvenience to himself. In his job he has the reputation of being most kind and supportive.

Ruthless—In business negotiations he is not adverse to subterfuge and intimidation to exact an outcome to his liking.

Violent, Sadistic and Explosive—While addicted to heroin he was involved in a number of brawls and fights and broke his hand on one occasion and sustained a number of other injuries and lacerations in other fights. On more than one occasion he brutally beat a pet cat to death because the cat scratched, disobeyed, or frustrated him. At work his executive director avoided him because of menacing, explosive confrontations.

Passive—Whatever dates or social contacts he had were usually at the initiative of friends and family. Despite his passivity, and probably because he is likeable, women at work ask him for dates and do favors for him. He spends many weekends alone watching T.V.

Active/Restless—He went out of his way at work to assume risky security responsibilities and functions. He has always been attracted to leisure activities and sports that are the most active, exciting, and dangerous. His hobbies barely sublimate his aggression. Although his drug involvement has often placed him on the other side of the law, he has always been intrigued with law enforcement activities and enjoyed his contact with law enforcement personnel. He recently took up martial arts.

Disavowal—He insists that he must be tough in his work or he will be considered a "patsy and soft." He has insisted that he can handle his loneliness and doesn't need companionship. Despite this he will often cruise in his car seeking a pickup. Recently and after much therapeutic work he now admits that he is worried less about rejection in asking for dates, but feels awkward and embarrassed to reveal his need and interest in companionship.

The need for satisfactions, shown in the patient described, is countered by a need to maintain psychological equilibrium and homeostasis. Such patients are in constant fear that their precarious equilibrium will be disrupted. Defenses that are commonly employed to maintain such an equilibrium include denial and disavowal. Passive longings and wishes are frequently defended against by activity and the defensive assumption of aggressive attitudes. To indulge wishes and wants is felt to be hazardous because one runs the risk of disappointment, frustration, rage, and narcissistic decompensation. Defenses are employed in the service of containing a whole range of longings and aspirations, but particularly those related to dependency and nurturance needs. It is because of massive repression of these needs that such individuals feel cut off, hollow and empty.

We suspect that addicts' inability to acknowledge and pursue actively their needs to be admired, and to love and be loved, leave them vulnerable to reversion to narcotic addiction on at least two counts. First of all, in failing to find suitable outlets for their needs, they fail to build up gradually a network of relationships, activities and involvements that act as buffers against boredom, depression, and narcissistic withdrawal; this latter triumvirate of affects acts powerfully to compel such individuals to use opiates. Furthermore, in failing to practice at expressing and changing their wants and needs, they are then subject to sporadic, uneven breakthroughs of their impulses and wishes in unpredictable and inappropriate ways that are often doomed to frustration and failure. The resulting rage and anger that grows out of such disappointment also compels a reversion to opiates.

TREATMENT IMPLICATIONS

We believe that effective treatment of narcotic addicts rests on more precisely identifying the underlying psychopathology and character disturbance. To do this requires the establishment of control over the addiction and the destructive activity and behavior often associated with it. However, this is understandably no easy task. The addict trusts his solutions more than ours. We also know that the use of drugs has played a most important part in regulating and controlling the addict's otherwise overwhelming anxiety, depression and rage. The challenge of initial treatment interventions is to provide acceptable provisions and substitutes for the drugs in order to create the structure and time that make understanding and management of the addict's problems possible. Briefly, our main allies for intervention and treatment remain the traditional institutions (courts, prisons, and hospitals), drug substitution (e.g., methadone maintenance, other psychoactive drugs) and human relationships. The specific ways in which we employ these interventions will be touched upon briefly in this discussion.

In many instances, institutional treatment will continue to be imposed, and in certain cases, required. Such options continue to be distasteful to most of us, but often necessary. As time goes on we may devise institutions that will avoid the extremes of prisons where there is too little understanding, and hospitals where there is perhaps too much understanding but insufficient controls. The balance of controls and understanding is essential for the management and treatment of behavioral problems.

Although we, and others, have advanced specific hypotheses that propose a psychological and physiologic basis for the clinical effectiveness of methadone maintenance, I suspect that one of the main benefits of methadone maintenance is the general control and internal chemical support the individual derives which then makes other human interventions possible. Methadone and other psychotropic drugs similarly have a generally "prosthetic" value and act as a benign chemical substitute for those used by our addicts.

As the available range of interventions helps to establish control over the malignant aspects of drug use, in subsequent phases of treatment we will be in a better position to identify and grapple with the specific impairments, vulnerabilities and characteristics of narcotic addicts. As we have already indicated, drug use and its attendant activities have substituted for defenses, relationships and other satisfactions. As this process is reversed with increasing control, the usual result is the emergence of underlying psychopathology and characterologic problems.

Some psychotherapeutic implications for these problems have already been hinted at. The necessity for consistency, empathy, activity and availability is apparent. Readiness to put into words the addict's feelings that he can hardly recognize or identify for himself, or others, is essential. Firm but non-punitive confrontation of violent and unacceptable behavior is also often required. The therapist must also be active in pointing out the patient's inability or disinclination to perceive danger and risk in his daily living.

The fragile to non-existent self-esteem in addicts must be appreciated continuously. Massive confrontations about their problems with violence and rage should be avoided. Similarly, passive longings and dependency problems should not be overexposed; defenses that serve to disguise such problems should be dealt with gingerly and respectfully. However, one should not ignore the destructive consequences and/or withdrawal when such defenses are extreme and exaggerated. I have found it useful to approach these problems gradually by identifying the difficulties around the inability of such patients to gain "sufficient satisfaction" out of life. This is done by repeatedly but tactfully identifying, whenever it comes up, the patient's tendencies to pursue extremes of indulgence or self-denial in relation to his wishes, relationships and activities. In the therapeutic relationship, extremes of aloofness or exaggerated friendliness are avoided by the therapist; questions are answered; sharing of personal experience and requests for practical assistance around daily living problems are again dealt with by avoiding extremes of withholding or giving. Generally, attempts are made to gradually help our patients overcome their exaggerated self-sufficiency and to see that they can overcome their fears and mistrust about involving themselves, and that the world can provide reasonable degrees of satisfaction.

Finally, some brief consideration about the use of psychoactive drugs seems pertinent. Clearly, addicts to some extent have known what is good for them. Had they not medicated themselves, many would not have survived or lived as well or as long as they did. It is surprising then to see how often psychotropic drugs are withheld and/or not considered in so many treatment programs. I believe that it is heroic and unrealistic to believe that we can reverse or resolve the enormous psychological damage and impairment in addicts through our psychotherapeutic interventions alone. We should be ready to consider flexibly the use of psychotropic drugs as an adjunct to psychotherapy, or as the primary therapy, depending on the assessment of the degree and nature of the addict's impairment, and a precise identification of target symptoms and affect states. Klein (1975) has recently reviewed psychopharmacological approaches to borderline states and strongly urges that we work to identify target symptoms better, with a particular emphasis on affect states. He also stresses the efficacy of matching specific types of antidepressants (e.g., MAO inhibitors vs. tricyclics) and phenothiazines to target symptoms and affect states, and the use of lithium for stabilizing affect swings and behavior. These are promising findings that are applicable to the understanding and treatment of narcotic addiction and warrant further study.

REFERENCES

Abraham, K. The psychological relation between sexuality and alcoholism. *Selected Papers of Karl Abraham.* New York: Basic Books, 1960.
Chein, I. et al. *The Road to H.* New York: Basic Books, 1964.
Fenichel, O. *The Psychoanalytic Theory of Neurosis.* New York: W.W. Norton, 1945.
Freud, S. Three essays on the theory of sexuality (1905). SE, Vol. 7. London: Hogarth Press, 1953.
Glover, E. On the etiology of drug addiction. *On the Early Development of Mind.* New York: Int. Univ. Press, 1956.
Kernberg, O.F. *Borderline Conditions and Pathological Narcissism.* New York: J. Aronson, Inc., 1975.
Khantzian, E.J. A preliminary dynamic formulation of the psychopharmacologic action of methadone. *Proc. Fourth National Methadone Conference, San Francisco,* January 1972.
———. Opiate addiction: A critique of theory and some implications for treatment. *Am J Psychother,* 28:59-70, 1974a.
———, Mack, J., and Schatzberg, A.F. Heroin use as an attempt to cope: Clinical observations. *Am J Psychiatry,* 131:160-164, 1974b.
———. Self selection and progression in drug dependence. *Psychiatry Digest,* 36:19-22, October 1975.

_____ and Kates, W. Group treatment of unwilling addicted patients: Programmatic and clinical aspects. *Int J Group Psychother*, 1976, in press.

Klein, D.F. Psychopharmacology and the borderline patient. *Borderline States in Psychiatry*. New York: Grune & Stratton, 1975.

Kohut, H. *The Analysis of the Self*. New York: Int. Univ. Press, 1971.

Krystal, H., and Raskin, H.A. *Drug Dependence. Aspects of Ego Functions*. Detroit: Wayne State Univ. Press, 1970.

Mahler, M.S. *On Human Symbiosis and the Viscissitudes of Individuation*. New York: Int. Univ. Press, 1968.

Meissner, W.W., Mack, J.E., and Semrad, E.V. Classical psychoanalysis. In: *Comprehensive Textbook of Psychiatry*. Freedman, A., Kaplan, H.I., and Sadock, B.J., eds. Baltimore: Williams & Wilkins, 1975.

Milkman, H., and Frosch, W.A. On the preferential abuse of heroin and amphetamine. *J Nerv Ment Dis*, 156:242-248, 1973.

Rado, S. The psychoanalysis of pharmacothymia. *Psychoanal Q*, 2:1-23, 1933.

_____. Narcotic bondage. A general theory of the dependence on narcotic drugs. *Am J Psychiatry*, 114:165-170, 1957.

Savit, R.A. Psychoanalytic studies on addiction: Ego structure in narcotic addiction. *Psychoanal Q*, 32:43-57, 1954.

Vaillant, G.E. Sociopathy as a human process. *Arch Gen Psychiatry*, 32:178-183, 1975.

Wieder, H., and Kaplan, E.H. Drug use in adolescents: psychodynamic meaning and pharmacogenic effect. *Psychoanal Study Child*, 24:399-431, 1969.

Wikler, A.A., and Rasor, R.W. Psychiatric aspects of drug addiction. *Am J Med*, 14:566-570, 1953.

Winnicott, D.W. Transitional objects and transitional phenomena. *Int J Psychoanal*, 34:89-97, 1953.

Wishnie, H. Opioid addiction: A masked depression. *Masked Depression*. S. Lesse, ed. New York: J. Aronson, Inc., 1974.

Wurmser, L. Psychoanalytic considerations of the etiology of compulsive drug use. *J Am Psychoanal Assoc*, 22:820-843, 1974.

Zinberg, N.E. Addiction and ego function. *Psychoanal Study Child*, 30:567-588, (T), 1975.

CHAPTER 8

Transference Phenomena in the Treatment of Addictive Illness: Love and Hate in Methadone Maintenance

Virginia Davidson, M.D.

INTRODUCTION

Wilfred Bion observed that "society, like the individual, may not want to deal with its stresses by psychological means until driven to do so by a realization that at least some of its distresses are psychological in origin" (Bion 1959). After more than a decade of experience in methadone maintenance, there is now widespread acknowledgment—even if it is belated, often grudging, and sometimes obscure—that attempts to treat heroin addiction by chemical means alone have failed. This admission of failure has crept stealthily into the literature, seemingly unnoticed at any given time because of the lack of emphasis on its presence. Terms such as "ancillary services," "social, personal, or vocational rehabilitation," and "supportive counseling" camouflage the fact that some meaningful psychological intervention has to take place in the treatment of addicted patients, or they will relapse to heroin use. Each time we read these phrases, we assume we know what they mean. They are as expectable by now, and are about as brief and meaningful as the complimentary close at the end of a business letter. Recent, typical examples from the March 1976 *Archives of General Psychiatry* include this statement from one author's summary about the effectiveness of the narcotic antagonists (Meyer et al. 1976):

Blocking drugs may be very usefully applied as *adjuncts* (italics mine) to psychologic intervention.

118

From another article (Goldstein 1976) in the same journal we learn that:

Alternative satisfactions have to be developed to substitute for those previously obtained from heroin. Experiences that are better and more satisfying than heroin use have to be built into a new behavioral repertoire. Self-image has to be improved, a new sense of worth has to be developed.

The author goes on to say that *without* this accomplishment, relapse to heroin use is virtually certain. Who with experience in treating addicts would disagree with such a sensible observation? Yet there is little in the literature of the treatment of the addictions which indicates that we understand what such claims imply about the necessity for accomplishing such massive personality change in addicted patients.

If the allegations are taken seriously that psychologic intervention will be necessary in conjunction with whatever chemical remedy is offered to treat addictive illness, it is curious that no coherent body of literature has developed that addresses the problems of psychologic treatment even after there is agreement that it is necessary.

Rather, the introduction of each new chemical is associated with an eagerness to discard the previous experience gained concerning the need for psychologic intervention, and hope emerges for a brief time that the new drug alone will produce a cure. This cycle has operated through the introduction of methadone, long-acting methadone, and each one of the narcotic antagonists, by turns. The wish to locate the cure for addictive illness *outside* the patient's psyche is obviously very strong in the persons who have been engaged in drug abuse research and treatment over the past 10 years. It probably exists in a stronger form only in the addicted patient him- or herself, where it is called "denial." Yet it is interesting to note that the same process exists in patients and researchers alike, though with perhaps varying degrees of intensity.

BACKGROUND

In this paper I shall describe certain recurring patterns of behavior which I observed in methadone maintenance patients during a 34-month period I worked in the setting of a methadone maintenance clinic. I shall relate these patterns to the descriptions in the psychoanalytic literature of ego defense mechanisms, and draw certain parallels between the behavior I observed in the clinic setting with the descriptions of transference phenomena which have been observed in the psychoanalysis of patients with so-called borderline personality organization (Kernberg 1975). Other writers, notably Khantzian, Mack, and Schatzberg (1974) and Vaillant (1975) have called attention to the primitive nature of the defenses in addicted patients. The defenses which Vaillant refers to as "immature"--splitting, denial, and projective identification—correspond to those which characterize patients with borderline personality organization, best described by Otto Kernberg (1975). Khantzian, in his study, notes an *absence* of neurotic defenses in his patients, but does not go on to describe the existence of more archaic patterns. Leon Wurmser (1974) has added much to the understanding of compulsive drug use by relating it to "narcissistic crises" in the lives of the individual drug abusers. Wurmser states that he has never seen a compulsive drug abuser who was not emotionally deeply disturbed, and he links this disturbance to the borderline type of psychopathology. In spite of observations such as these by persons who have had considerable experience in treating addicted patients in individual psychotherapy, most of the psychological treatment of addicts will be left to those persons in the treatment hierarchy who have the least knowledge and experience in psychotherapy. There are no serious attempts to gain—for addicts—access to the best forms of psychotherapy available, partly because of the process that involves denying that addictive illness has psychological origins, but also because of the extremely trying nature of therapy with borderline patients (Leibovich 1975; Pines 1975), even if they are not addicted to heroin.

TRANSFERENCE PHENOMENA AND COUNTERTRANSFERENCE BEHAVIOR

Transference is a term which implies that the patient's behavior at a given moment in treatment is determined more by his very early experiences with significant others than by the reality stimulus of the present setting.

I use the term transference phenomena to refer to observable patterns of behavior in patients' transactions with clinic staff members and the clinic itself, as well as in their relationships with individual therapists. Whenever there are rapid shifts in the way patients perceive others, whenever strong affective states such as love or hatred are predominant (and especially when there is rapid alternation between the two), and whenever there is a powerful projection of hostile, aggressive impulses from the patient to someone else, it is safe to say that transference phenomena are present. These responses I have just described are not perceived by the patient as being unusual or strange, in fact they are natural for him or her, and characterize the styles of relating to others that he/she has developed from early life.

Countertransference, as used in this paper, will refer to the totality of the therapist's response to the patient. It includes reality factors such as the setting and the working alliance with the patient, plus the internal response of the therapist to the patient.

CHARACTERISTIC PATTERNS OF BEHAVIOR IN THE CLINIC AND RELATED MANAGEMENT PROBLEMS

The behavior of methadone patients in the clinic setting is remarkable in several respects, when compared with the behavior of other groups of psychiatric patients whose treatment utilizes the outpatient clinic format. I shall focus on three major observable differences in the clinic behavior of methadone patients, and comment on the kinds of difficulties each one presents for staff management in the outpatient methadone maintenance clinic. I believe that these patterns of behavior are roughly equivalent to the ego defense mechanisms of splitting, projective identification, and denial, which have been described in the psychoanalytic literature dealing with the treatment of borderline patients (Kernberg 1975), even though the behavior described is occurring in the context of an outpatient clinic.

1. Analogous to splitting are *manifestations in the clinic setting of extreme affects*, which appear to be inappropriate to the reality stimulus of the moment. These affective states are usually characterized by extreme rage; for example, murderous hatred can be expressed by a patient toward a dispensing nurse who does not ready the medication as soon as the patient expects it. This expression of rage is limited to the situation in which it emerged—the patient does not carry the feeling over to everyone else he/she encounters. Feelings of contrition and remorse are likely to follow closely the expression of hatred and rage. What is familiar to workers in methadone is the rapidity with which patients can oscillate between extreme states of feeling. The patient has diminished capacity to modulate feelings, so must swing back and forth between strong positive and strong negative affects.

Problems for staff in relating to this aspect of the addicted patient's personality are enormous. Expression of strong hostility, anger, and blamefulness in patients arouses equally powerful emotions in staff, whose most common response is to retaliate—overtly or covertly—against the patient. In physicians, this is most commonly expressed through the dosage of methadone, since this is the powerful medium through which most patient contacts occur. All of us know patients who manage to alienate the staff one by one, then find themselves removed from the program for violations of one sort or another. The staff is usually not aware of this process, and will deny—if asked—feeling hostility and suppressed rage toward the patient. In a well-run program this process of retaliation against the patient can be minimized by enlightened supervision, ideally by someone *outside* the treatment system.

Related to retaliation as a means of coping with the patient's tendency to experience strong emotions separately and intensely (splitting), is pairing. Patients "select" a staff member with whom they establish a dependent, demanding, and clinging relationship. Few negative emotions are channeled into this relationship, but rather are expressed in strong dislikes for and refusals to deal with other staff. The "chosen" staff person becomes the patient's advocate in all matters relating to progress and performance, and may at times jealously protect the patient from having contact with other staff. While patient-staff pairing is less destructive than retaliation, in that it allows some patients to remain in treatment through thick and thin, it cannot be therapeutic for the patient unless it carries some generalizability to other relationships. As long as the therapist is obtaining gratification from the "specialness" of the relationship, this is not likely to occur.

2. Analogous to projective identification is the *expectation on the part of patients that they will be unfairly dealt with by treatment personnel, and an associated tendency to perceive the external environment as hostile and threatening,* regardless of what the actual circumstances are. Because of the fact that addicts live dangerous lives in their search for drugs, and because they are frequently incarcerated or are being implicated in criminal activities, we assume it is reasonable for them to behave in a suspicious, guarded, and untrusting manner when they come to treatment. While this kind of explanation might possibly account for the addict's initial problems in relating to the staff, it cannot begin to account for the persistent incapacities in forming trusting relationships that exist for years after the patient has begun treatment.

For any staff, the task of providing the qualities that are necessary for a therapeutic alliance to be established with the patient is difficult when the patient's problems are manifest in qualities that appear to make this primary task impossible. Staff members, to be effective, must maintain the capacity to be empathic toward the patient; the patient, however, behaves in such a way toward "helping" people that this empathic quality in staff is always undermined and jeopardized. All therapists must maintain a sense of their own worth and value; they must have self-esteem and a sense that the work they do with patients "matters." Yet when the patient's style of relating involves projecting onto others the intensely aggressive, hostile, and negative impulses felt inside, the other person (in this case, the therapist) receives constant messages that he/she is being aggressive, hostile, and unsympathetic toward the patient. In my experience, most methadone patients are not capable of distinguishing the origin of these hostile impulses except after years of exposure to a person who can remain relatively neutral in the face of these sorts of accusations.

With therapeutic problems of this magnitude, not to become locked into an equally hostile countertransference relationship is a monumental task for the best-trained and most talented of therapists; for the untrained, unskilled, and uninitiated, it is virtually impossible.

3. *Denial of entire segments of reality, especially involving behavior concerning drug usage* is typical; related forms of denial are evident in the need patients demonstrate to appear impervious to the impact methadone maintenance has on their lives. Patients commonly express the belief that *they* are in control of their drug usage —they maintain that they will be able to withdraw from methadone at a future time of their own choosing, even after previous attempts have resulted in quick relapse to heroin. Years of compulsive drug use have not altered the psychic reality of many patients—namely, disbelief in the reality of the psychologic component of their addictive illness. Denial of feelings of anxiety and depression in addicted patients has been discussed by other writers (Vaillant 1975), as well as the return of these feelings during attempted withdrawal from methadone and the necessity for psychological support during withdrawal (Chappel et al. 1973; Lowinson and Langrod 1973). Denial, in the psychological sense, is most often confused by staff with conscious lying and manipulation. While addicted patients certainly have in common with other patients the habits of lying and manipulation, it is impressive to what extent the latter explanations are used by staff members to account for patients' behavior.

The gruff, loud, and complaining behavior that patients exhibit toward appointments often covers up the desperate fear these patients have about emotional contact with another person. Their apparent superficial involvement in counseling is often interpreted by staff as "low motivation." Grumbling about having to keep appointments, complaints about the time lost in the clinic, and especially assertions that the counseling relationship is a waste of time, may mask the patient's terror of involvement. Many times I have had the experience of hearing vituperative protests from patients that keeping their appointment with me would cause them to be fired from the job; that they simply could not afford the time to discuss their medication, and so on. Yet these same patients, once in the office, shed their belligerence like an unwanted skin, and want to discuss more than their medication. So what masquerades as a devil-may-care attitude toward the clinic frequently represents massive denial of the importance of the clinic in the patient's life. Sometimes only during withdrawal from methadone does this attachment to the clinic enter the patient's awareness.

CONCLUSION

By describing typical patterns of behavior that can be observed in methadone maintenance patients in the outpatient clinic setting, I have attempted to demonstrate that this behavior is markedly different from that observed in other groups of psychiatric patients who are treated in outpatient clinics. Much of the "difficult" behavior is often seen as part of a constellation of undesirable social characteristics attributed to addicted patients. Staff may try to eradicate this behavior (usually through elaboration and enforcement of clinic rules) with the associated hope that the patient will become more compliant, and then amenable to therapy. This is somewhat akin to stating that if the patient did not have psychological problems he/she would be easier to treat.

I am suggesting that the behavior we see in the patient *is* the manifestation of his/her problems in living, and not an artifact of either the clinic setting or of the addicted patient's sociocultural background. This behavior makes sense, so to speak, if it is related to the ego defense mechanisms which have been delineated in the psychoanalytic study of borderline patients. The problems which this behavior presents for the outpatient psychotherapy of addicted patients are considerable, as I have attempted to show, and are similar to the problems encountered whenever the treatment of any borderline patient is undertaken. Understanding why (and when) patients establish negative transferences can lead to effective management, and to the prevention of transference psychoses, which are not infrequent in this population of patients. It is crucial to protect and nurture the positive transference relationships that develop; for many patients it is easier first to establish a positive bond with the clinic than with a counselor. Whenever clinics are structured in such a way that this is an unreasonable expectation, treatment prospects remain glum.

REFERENCES

Bion, W. *Experiences in Groups*. New York: Basic Books, 1959. p. 22.

Chappel, J., Skolnick, V., and Senay, E. Techniques of withdrawal from methadone and their outcome over six months to two years. *Proceedings of the 5th National Conference on Methadone Treatment*, Washington, D.C., 1973. pp. 482-489.

Goldstein, A. Heroin addiction. *Arc Gen Psychiatry*, 33(3):353-358, 1976.

Jackman, J. A hypothesis concerning the difficulty of withdrawal from maintenance of methadone. *Proceedings of the 5th National Conference on Methadone Treatment*, Washington, D.C., 1973. pp. 471-475.

Kernberg, O. *Borderline Conditions and Pathological Narcissism*. New York: Jason Aronson, 1975.

Khantzian, E., Mack, J., and Schatzberg, A. Heroin use as an attempt to cope: Clinical observations. *Am J Psychiatry*, 131(2):160-164, 1974.

Leibovich, M. An aspect of the psychotherapy of borderline personalities. *Psychother Psychosom*, 25:53-57, 1975.

Lowinson, J., and Langrod, J. Detoxification of long-term methadone patients. *Proceedings of the 5th National Conference on Methadone Treatment*, Washington, D.C., 1973. pp. 256-261.

Meyer, R., Mirin, S., Altman, J., and McNamee, B. A behavioral paradigm for the evaluation of narcotic antagonists. *Arch Gen Psychiatry*, 33:371-377, 1976.

Pines, M. Borderline personality organization. *Psychother Psychosom*, 25:58-62, 1975.

Vaillant, G. Sociopathy as a human process. *Arch Gen Psychiatry*, 32:178-183, 1975.

Wurmser, L. Psychoanalytic considerations of the etiology of compulsive drug use. *J Am Psychoanal Assoc*, 22:4, 820-843, 1974.

CHAPTER 9

Implications of Psychodynamics for Therapy in Heroin Use: A Borderline Case

Eugene H. Kaplan, M.D.

Psychoanalytic formulations began with the psychoneuroses. Freud subsequently studied more severe disturbances as well, developing his theories of narcissism and the psychoses (Freud 1957a, 1957b). The scope has expanded to embrace the whole gamut of mental conditions, with the ultimate goal to make psychoanalysis a general psychology (Loewenstein et al. 1966). At the same time, the progressive refinements in theoretical conceptualization have permitted increasing precision in defining psychopathology in terms of id, ego and superego functions and malfunctions.

The early psychoanalytic literature emphasized the instinctual drive component of drug abuse (Yorke 1970). Interdependent advances in clinical observation and theory have equipped us better to study heroin users. Pfeiffer has reviewed the evolution of the concept of the borderline states (1975). In 1942, Deutsch described "as-if" personalities. Psychoanalytic treatment showed the common thread of an impoverished emotionality different from the schizophrenic, with widely different symptom pictures (1942). Hoch and Polatin (1949) reported on a group of patients who showed both neurotic and psychotic features, but were classifiable as neither. In Schmideberg's view, this group bordered not only on neurosis and psychosis, but on psychopathy and normality as well (1959). Grinker's research team found multiple, shifting psychological defense mechanisms in hospitalized borderline patients (1968). Grinker considered this shifting combination of neurotic, psychotic, psychopathic and normal defense mechanisms to typify borderline

126

patients. Using the theoretical framework of psychoanalytic ego psychology and following Knight's suggestions, he assessed ego functions systematically (1953). Grinker concluded that the borderline syndrome is characterized by the arrested development of ego functions.

Summarizing some salient features of the borderline syndrome will make it clear why many heroin users are classifiable in this diagnostic rubric (Pavenstedt 1967; Minuchin et al. 1967):

(1) Intractable mistrust and suspiciousness, with a predisposition for transient paranoid psychotic episodes.

(2) Stunted cognitive capacity, fixated on concrete thinking, with relatively little abstract conceptualization. This leads to an inability to profit from past experience, to look ahead to the future.

(3) Intense self-centeredness and preoccupation with need-satisfaction, with obliviousness to the rights, needs and desires of others. These traits seriously interfere with personal relationships, which tend to be brief and manipulative, or markedly dependent and ambivalent. The other person is viewed as a supplier of needs, an obstruction to need-gratification, or a danger.

(4) Fluidity and insufficient demarcation of self-boundaries. The intense dependent relationships (which might appear to contradict the feature of egocentricity), often involve such fluid self-boundaries. The other person is viewed not as a separate and distinct entity, but as part of the self. This can lead to catastrophic separation reactions.

(5) Self-esteem is highly volatile, and exquisitely dependent on external sources rather than inner resources.

(6) Self-control is poor and dependent on cues and signals from external sources. Control emanates from others rather than from internalized norms and values.

Points 5 and 6 indicate that, despite the self-centeredness, overall mental functioning is characterized by disequilibrium resulting from an inability to rely on oneself.

(7) Emotions tend to be strong and primitive, "all-or-nothing," without nuances and refinements, and heavily laden with hostility and aggression.

(8) Many of the above contribute to the proclivity to impulsive action.

The number of chronic heroin users who have been psychoanalyzed is very small. To these data, we may add the clinical findings of psychoanalytically trained observers working with such patients in other settings. While statistical studies of the mass treatment programs deserve careful scrutiny, Stoller argues compellingly for the heuristic usefulness of the individual case history:

> . . . the intensively studied single case has given way to the more rapidly observed many. There is certainly good reason for this: extravagant conclusions have frequently been drawn from a single case; at times these conclusions have not even followed from the data collected. Moreover, it has often been impossible to be sure what were actually data and what was conjecture. These difficulties have led to the present emphasis on controlled studies with adequate samples. Not only does the researcher thus conform more to the standards of science but he also renders his activity less painful . . . he reduces his involvement with his subjects' distress . . . and he avoids the sense of uncertainty that besets the clinician in his one-to-one relationship with his patient.
>
> Yet, although statistical techniques may enable us to corroborate or deny a hypothesis, they do not produce one. On the other hand, as Freud's work shows, the extended case study is an inexhaustible source of ideas. Unhappily, those of us who are clinicians, especially psychoanalysts, seem to have little feel or need for proper controls and checks on reliability, whereas those who like their facts "hard" too often deny the depths and complexities of mental functioning and thus avoid the excitement and uncertainty that facing them entails (Stoller 1973, pp. x-xi).

Sally Y is a 25-year-old white single upper-middle-class woman diagnosed as borderline by at least four psychiatrists.[1] In 5 years, her intravenous heroin use escalated from occasional to weekend to Type III escape (Wieder and Kaplan 1969), two to five bags daily. A drug user of the Type III category is defined as one who "takes drugs to escape the severe suffering of a chronically painful ego state."

When the Y's first consulted me, it was not about Sally. She had recovered from an acute psychotic episode some 18 months before, precipitated by prolonged severe abuse of methaqualone and LSD. Since then, Sally was living in a remote corner of the country, apparently self-supporting and functioning, and the Y's seemed relieved at the outcome. In the aftermath of Sally's decompensa-

---

[1]This report is based on the author's 3½-year psychotherapy of her parents, Mr. and Mrs. Y, consultative evaluations of Sally and her sister, and ongoing coordinating discussions with Sally's present psychiatrist, Arthur M. Schwartz, M.D., who has treated her for a year and a half.

tion, however, Mrs. Y complained that "our family is falling apart from depression."

Her complaint narrowed down to a lack of emotional support from her husband. I took him into thrice-weekly psychotherapy with rationale that any improvement in Mr. Y's impoverished object-relationships would redound to his wife's benefit as well. Mr. Y is a controlling, unfeeling, obsessive-narcissistic character beneath a smiling, easygoing facade. He readily admitted his avoidance of any close, giving relationship, which stemmed from a fear of being engulfed: "Give them a finger and they'll want the whole arm."

Part of his avoidance derived from early experiences with his unempathetic borderline mother who had raised him by the book. Whenever he had turned to his mother for understanding and support in childhood, her response was an admonitory lecture on etiquette tangential to his immediate problem, with punishments adding to his woes. His remote, narcissistic father was away "on business" months at a time, and showed little interest when home.

Both Mr. Y's parents were pathologically stingy. When he married, they rendered a bill for room and board since age 21 and for the engagement party they had tendered. Mr. Y reacted to their pathological parsimony with a combination . of material over-generosity and affectional stinginess. He supports his only sibling, a younger brother. Mr. Y's brother is a chronic drug abuser with paranoid trends who hasn't worked in 10 years. We were to learn later that Mr. Y's relationship with his brother was a prototype for that with Sally.

Mr. Y hardly ever spoke of Sally, but after a year in therapy, asked that I advise his wife about their daughter. Through these consultations with Mrs. Y, it became clear to me that Sally was probably reinvolved in chronic severe drug abuse. Furthermore, Mr. Y not only denied her involvement, but abetted it. Encouraging Sally's phone calls to his office, Mr. Y sent her money without out Mrs. Y's knowledge.

Where Mr. Y used denial and avoidance and underreacted, his wife is a pessimistic worrier who overacts with panic and self-blame. She is an infantile, dependent woman who herself suffered from maternal deprivation. She yearns for stability and security because of childhood experiences with a long succession of housekeepers and frequent moves all over the country. Mrs. Y never completed an academic year in one school until her teens. Mrs. Y's mother immersed herself in the family business, but periodically her neglect alternated with a self-centered need to mother without regard for her child's (Mrs. Y's) needs. This immature, narcissistic, clinging grandmother dominated her daughter and the grandfather with hysterical outbursts indistinguishable from tyrannizing temper tantrums.

When Mrs. Y married, she aspired to create the ideal family she fantasied in childhood. Instead, she recreated the relationship with her own mother, first with Mr. Y, then with Sally. Lacking self-esteem and devoid of any sense of entitlement, Mrs. Y asks: "Who am I to want anything for myself? Who am I to stand in the way of their desires and happiness?" This couple's neurotic needs mesh, for Mr. Y's attitude is one of dominating helpless entitlement. He expects Mrs. Y to be at his beck and call: "She has nothing better to do." In effect, she is his buffer, insulating him from the world by carrying out his commands. Mr. Y's attitude is that of the young child who deals with the threat of the loss of his sense of magic omnipotence in the course of separation-individuation. Delegating this power to the now separate mother, he yet retains anal-sadistic domination of her.

Mr. Y is unable to purchase his own clothes or to select what to wear in the morning. Mrs. Y must purchase and lay out his complete ensemble daily. She must attend to all the practical realities of everyday life. Mr. Y never has refueled the car nor had it serviced; he has never been in a department store or a hardware store. Yet Mr. Y knows what has to be done, daily preparing long lists of chores for Mrs. Y, his imperial ambassador to the outside world. Mrs. Y never objected, because in truth, she didn't know what to do with herself. Whenever her wifely and motherly duties were complete, she retired to bed to read or daydream, content. At once, she was the obedient little girl and the perfect all-giving wife and mother for which that little girl had yearned.

Sally's breakdown and hospitalization while at college shattered Mrs. Y's contentment. Robbed of her illusion of motherly perfection, she was wracked with self-blame. Furthermore, Mr. Y's emotional unavailability became so glaring that she could deny it no longer. For just as he refused all dealings with merchants, gardeners and auto repair men, he would have nothing to do with the hospital and the doctors. Of course, he was very interested, and would make lists of questions for Mrs. Y to ask the doctors, but the demands of his business precluded his personal involvement.

When Mrs. Y tearfully reproached him, Mr. Y would angrily accuse her of overreacting, minimize Sally's predicament, and present a list of social obligations she had neglected during the hospitalization. So I came to understand Mr. Y's willingness to have his wife consult me about Sally. When he could no longer deny her problem, he sought to avoid it in customary fashion, by delegation to Mrs. Y.

Once Sally was brought to my attention, I rapidly inferred both her serious drug involvement (without any certainty of heroin use) and her marked dependency on her parents. However, Mr. Y would deny the former and Mrs. Y was fearfully loathe to exercize the leverage this dependency implied. Therefore, it took 6 months more before the Y's could bring themselves to insist that Sally return home. Finally convinced that her financial dependence reflected a profound emotional dependence upon them, the Y's nevertheless were surprised at her easy compliance with their summons home. The pattern was repeated in the 4 additional months they took to insist upon her consulting me. Though guarded in the interview, Sally accepted my referral for psychotherapy with alacrity.

Mrs. Y had placed Sally in nursery school at 3 because she was having a rough pregnancy. Sally cried a great deal, and her mother often let her stay home. In subsequent years, the crying gave way to complaints of sore throats and "swollen glands." Though Mrs. Y was well aware that Sally's complaints had no physical basis, she could not insist that the child attend school those days.

Sally's only sibling, a sister 3 years younger, manifested a severe behavior disorder from age 2 to 6, with hyperactivity, hairpulling and trichophagia. During this 4-year period, 5 through 9, the mother feels that Sally was seriously neglected. From 7 to 11, Sally was treated for asthma, receiving weekly allergy shots and oral and intramuscular medication for acute attacks.

After a series of asthmatic attacks at summer camp at age 11, the parents were summoned. In their presence, the camp doctor accused Sally of bringing the attacks on, and told her to say so directly if she wished to go home. Mrs. Y was impelled to state that she would never force Sally to remain. Confronted thus, Sally chose to stay, suffering no further attacks.

Taking courage from the doctor's example, her parents offered Sally the dog long withheld on the basis of strong positive allergy tests. Sally agreed to the proviso that the dog would be taken away if she had another attack. None followed, and she's had a dog ever since.

According to her mother, Sally was a depressed, sluggish, unenthusiastic isolate from early childhood. Mrs. Y was always arranging for other children to come over and play. Left to herself, Sally ate candy and watched television, while the phone hardly ever rang. At 12, however, she went to a new camp. During the several summers there, she was enthusiastic and a model of responsibility, especially in caring for younger children. Sally got along well with the staff also, but her peer relations remained poor. Once back home, she reverted to sluggish isolation. Sally's habit of lying on her bed for hours in a reverie appeared around this time. Although Mrs. Y had long done the same, she had Sally checked several times for hypothyroidism.

Mrs. Y contrasts her two daughters. With her younger daughter, she always knows where she stands, for Mrs. Y's demands will be met with either anger or compliance. Sally's evasive indirection and withdrawal, however, make her mother exceedingly anxious. This is not only in response to Mrs. Y's demands, moreover. In her transference behavior, Sally exudes helpless neediness nonverbally, implicitly expecting the other to decode and supply her wants.

Once in her teens, Sally flouted family rules, driving without a license and ignoring curfews. Father denied the defiance while mother was paralyzed into fearful ineffectuality. They nevertheless took heart in Sally's cracking her shell of isolation and withdrawal in ninth grade. Unfortunately these peer relationships were, and continue to be, based on drug abuse. Such relationships, based on a shared activity or interest, rather than a genuine interest in the other person, are characteristic of early or pre-latency peer relationships.

As she prepared for college, Sally dealt with her separation anxiety. At summer orientation, she met a boy and quickly made arrangements to live with him. When this agreement fell through in the fall, Sally immediately found a replacement with whom she lived for over 2 years. Ned was a campus drug dealer who supplied her first heroin. He slept with a gun under the bed and was mortally afraid of needles. Yet, Sally found snorting unsatisfying compared to the intravenous route. Beginning with a sense of entitlement and self-reward, she enjoyed the excitement of setting up the works and flushing the blood back and forth in the syringe.

Heroin use was only occasional at this time, yet Sally's preference for "downs"—methaqualone, diazepam, chlordiazepoxide and barbiturates (Tuinal)—has been consistent. She found no pleasure or relief from "ups," and psychedelics made her fear losing control.

Sally began to decompensate at the beginning of her third college year. She was under greater stress as her studies became more rigorous, and her parents were increasing their criticism of her relationship with Ned. At first she visited a psychologist at home on weekends, and then entered analysis five times weekly in her college town. Soon she became fragmented, regressed and depressed.

After 6 weeks in a psychiatric hospital, which diagnosed her as a borderline personality with severe drug abuse, Sally spent 6 months at home, receiving once weekly supportive psychotherapy. For the next 2½ years, she led a subsidized hippie existence, dependent on "downs" and gradually increasing heroin use. Whenever money ran short, she called father collect at the office, making her requests palatable by citing the needs of her organic food or pottery-making business. By the time she returned home again and entered psychotherapy, Sally was physically dependent on heroin. Sally formed a dependent transference, and has not missed more than two sessions in 18 months. She comes a few minutes late to avoid waiting, wearing her coat, and carrying a tote bag with oral supplies—cigarettes, gum and candy. With the therapist's first absence, Sally signaled her exquisite intolerance of separation and the quick shift to another need-satisfying object. She had to leave on vacation first, so as not to be the one left behind. Before her psychiatrist returned, Sally confessed her heroin use to her parents for the first time.

Sally's confession was less a plea for help in stopping heroin than a response to her loss of oral supplies. She was flat broke. On Sally's return from hippiedom, Mrs. Y had taken over as in childhood, finding Sally an apartment and a roommate and paying the rent. Sally had made her own revisions quietly, moving in with a new-found boyfriend, a chronic heroin user of her own class and background. When everything had been expended for their combined habits, Sally turned to her parents. To get back home that day, she literally had to comb through her pockets for nickels and dimes to buy a couple of gallons of gas.

Sally remained abstinent for about one month, but her boyfriend's success in completing his studies and entering business pierced her formidable narcissism. Moreover, Sally very likely felt a separation threat, in fearing that his success would make him less needful of her. The blow to her omnipotent wishes and fragile self-esteem made her envious and resentful, and Sally reinitiated the mutual seduction with heroin. Soon, she was using five bags daily, and requiring two to "get off." After the boyfriend's business capital, a gift from his parents, was expended for heroin, Sally embezzled several thousands of dollars.

Mrs. Y had become alarmed by her daughter's more obvious episodes of somnolence, neglect of her responsibilities and abuse of family charge accounts. I drew the conclusion for Mrs. Y that the patient must have relapsed and that her earlier confession amounted to a plea for their intervention. Mrs. Y needed massive therapeutic support to withstand her daughter's evasiveness, lying and vituperative rage when accused. Mr. Y characteristically denied and disappeared. The mother lied to me in turn, claiming falsely that she had canceled all her charge accounts. Finally, the exposure of Sally's embezzlements overcame Mr. Y's denial, and the parents painfully implemented my recommendation for hospitalization.

Sally offered no significant opposition and withdrawal was accomplished easily. Threats of and reactions to separation pervaded this period, with Sally seeking to control her parents' visits. If they came, she was withdrawn or belligerent; if they asked to come, she rejected them; but if they threatened not to visit, she pleaded for their presence.

The physician in charge of the detoxification unit proceeded with family therapy despite his knowledge of the preexisting therapeutic arrangements. He told the assembled family that they all shared the blame for Sally's addiction. The validity of his statement was vitiated by his style and timing. Her sister was consumed with guilt. When I had seen the sister over a year before, she had described her closeness and loyalty which kept her from revealing Sally's drug involvement to their parents. Her guilt was reinforced by sibling rivalry. In reaction to Sally's first breakdown, sister consciously resolved to become the opposite, rejecting the drug-using long-hairs, and becoming the studious athlete. The motivation was not only fear of drugs, but the wish to please the Y's and prove that they were not total failures as parents. Already mother's favorite, she also was trying unsuccessfully to dislodge Sally from her preferred status with father.

Parenthetically, the sister's need to please her parents and fulfill their aspirations was linked with a marked identity problem. She didn't know how much she did to fulfill her own wishes, how much the wishes of others. Sister hates to feel lazy and is compelled to keep busy, suggestive of a struggle against that to which Sally has surrendered. Sister's drug preferences reflect this struggle. In contrast to Sally, sister dislikes marihuana and prefers amphetamines, for Type II coping: "I have a disorganized mind and go off on tangents. Speed concentrates it and I do much better studying and on exams."

Detoxification completed, Sally was transferred to another hospital where her therapist was completely in charge of her treatment. The first weekend after the transfer, Mrs. Y made a suicide attempt with sleeping pills after Mr. Y went off on a business trip in the face of her bitter objections. I did not hospitalize Mrs. Y after her emergency room visit. In the next 2 weeks, she responded to small doses of Navane as an antidepressant, and to interpretations of her dependency.

I told Mrs. Y that she tried to satisfy her own intense dependency needs and fear of abandonment vicariously, through being the ever-dependable satisfier of everyone else's needs. She took care of the family as she wished to be taken care of. Mrs. Y's severe insomnia, symptomatic of her depression, abated for the first time in

5 years. (Five years before Sally had been hospitalized, the maternal grandmother had suffered a nervous breakdown, and the maternal uncle had suicided.)

Mrs. Y's responses to the interpretations also emphasized dependency and separation: "I had only two models for marriage—my mother who clung to my father 24 hours a day, except once a week when she got all her mothering in on me . . . and the perfect marriage of my uncle who lived around the corner. He treated his wife as his sister (Mrs. Y's mother) wanted to be treated—'til one day, after 25 years, he hung himself. All my mothering came from maids, and they had to mother my mother, too . . . I feel as if my motor has been restarted." For the first time ever, Mrs. Y then made independent plans for a weekend.

In her therapy sessions, Sally seems to be asking to be given, told, fed, without directly asking. If her doctor is slow to respond, she flushes, verges on tears, and asks how long before she'll feel better. Her enthusiasm and energy seem to run down within 10 minutes, and her chronic dissatisfaction mounts. She gets angry and by the end of the session seems sleepy. Sally chain smokes cigarettes and chews gum throughout.

The therapist came early every morning with coffee and cake until Sally's weight gain (at least 15 lbs. in 2 months) became obvious. Sally seemed happy about the discipline when the cake was discontinued. Discussions of her weight gain have led to associations about her sister, suggesting not only the rivalry with the lithe and muscular sister but also identification with the mother withdrawn and self-preoccupied during the pregnancy with sister.

After detoxification, Sally received Triavil 4-25 *qid*, since reduced to 2-25, and gradually progressed to working during the day and returning to the hospital at night. With each increment of freedom she tested the limits: returning intoxicated from marihuana, smuggling in marihuana, refusing to attend the compulsory patient meetings. Her therapist stressed that every wish she has ever expressed at home has been gratified. Firm and distinct limits are required so she can gradually learn to tolerate frustration, for which she is praised. Sally's relationship with the therapist seems shallow and without curiosity, but the therapeutic alliance has endured.

Sally was able to join her parents for long weekends several times since her hospitalization. Each time the mother extended the weekend without notice, encroaching upon the therapy sessions. This seems to repeat in microcosm Mrs. Y's bitter childhood experience of being pulled out of school every year to accompany her parents so that she never completed an academic year in one place. For the first time, Sally was able to refuse their invitation, stating that therapy had to come first. They felt compelled to leave her over $50 in cash. Before they left, the therapist reviewed the reactions she could anticipate. Though it was her own choice, Sally felt deserted nevertheless and acted out. She entered her grandparents' vacant apartment and took a hypodermic syringe and needle, but told her therapist about it. In libidinal terms, Sally's craving for heroin is on an oral level of fixation. Sally's oral problems began with infantile colic, and the tendency to overeat was well established by latency. Sally's aggressive orality is easily discernible in her voracious overeating and marked weight gain, her habit of constantly chewing ice, her blistering vituperative cursing when angered, and the oral attitudes of entitlement. Stealing is experienced as taking what she needs and therefore what she should have.

The orality is a necessary but insufficient determinant of Sally's drug use. The specific effects of heroin in enhancing her preexisting defense of withdrawal into reverie make it sought after for Type III use. So far, Sally has made it clear that heroin helps her surmount rage, oral envy and some ill-defined sexual impulses. In addition, heroin is used when she has a strong sense of entitlement and self-reward for accomplishment.

Although Sally dislikes the amphetamine "high," she uses them infrequently, in a Type II coping pattern. When Sally makes plans, she is very enthusiastic. As she encounters painful reality in attempting to implement her plans, her oral attitudes of entitlement and magical omnipotence are painfully unfulfilled and her fragile self-esteem crumbles. Frustration, rage and depression mount, and she may seek desperately to recapture activity magically through amphetamines, to accomplish her goal effortlessly.

Identification with mother is very evident in this regard. Mother has been unable to commit herself seriously to any activity outside of the house. Her reaction to any challenge is to feel threatened and to withdraw gracefully before she fails. So mother's days have been spent in limited volunteer and community activities; the few hours Mrs. Y spends in bed with a book almost every morning or afternoon are the prototype of the patient's reverie. Mother's fear of failure is most prominent in her overinvolvement with Sally; her self-esteem goes up and down with the ups and downs of Sally's condition.

Both Sally and her mother share the lack of a reservoir for self-esteem and resolve, requiring a constant oral inflow of support, direction and encouragement. Recently Sally was galvanized into registering for a specialized course by pressure from Mrs. Y and her sister. Immediately, she hoped that the course would be canceled.

After the first class, Sally dealt with her sense of abysmal ineffectuality by raging at her fellow students, questioning the usefulness of the course, and then fell into a deep undrugged sleep in her office for over 2 hours.

It is a commonplace report from abstinent drug abusers that they have experienced subjectively the drugged state while under stress. In Sally's case at least, this is more than an evocation of the wished-for drugged state. It is a continuation of a regressive withdrawal maneuver traceable back to her childhood. The next day, a progressive sequence similarly traceable to a childhood prototype could be discerned. Mrs. Y, borrowing courage from me as she had from the camp doctor many years ago, presented Sally with the necessity for a clear-cut choice. If the course was too much for her, it had to be dropped immediately lest several hundred dollars of tuition be forfeited. Sally chose to continue, and the past repeated itself; after passing the course with flying colors, Sally rewarded herself with a genuine heroin nod.

COMPARISON OF SALLY AND CLARA

The contributions to the clarification of borderline conditions from Kernberg, Mahler, Masterson and others have been most useful in understanding Sally and her parents. Her treatment has been based on this understanding. As Kernberg puts it, the diagnosis of borderline personality organization involves descriptive, structural and genetic-dynamic considerations. Assessment of the character pathology delineates the level and nature of instinctual development, superego development, defensive operations of the ego, and the vicissitudes of internalized object relationships (1968). In this metapsychological diagnostic context, Sally's heroin abuse is a facet of failure of resolution of the separation-individuation process typical of borderlines. She is an incomplete person, unable to maintain self-regulation. Her psychological homeostasis requires an attachment to external objects to supplement the structural defects; in Sally's case, the objects include drugs as well as people.

It must be emphasized, however, that borderline personality organization is not invariably associated with drug abuse. The importance of a detailed diagnostic assessment is illustrated by comparing Sally with Clara, another 25-year-old borderline woman who is terrified of drugs. While Sally manifests direct and unrestrained gratification of her fixation at the oral level, Clara shows evidence of incomplete advances to higher libidinal stages. Clara's significant oral, anal and negative oedipal fixations are defended against by a constant, fearful preoccupation with losing control.

Both patients were overweight children. Sally reacts with oral envy of her younger sister; Clara has always protested loudly and successfully against parental attention directed to her younger brother and sister, and insists on the choicest morsel of any food. In early adolescence, Sally's oral indulgence extended to drugs; drug satiation curbed her desire to eat, enabling her to lose some weight. At the same developmental milestone, Clara unveiled severe primitive defenses against her oral impulses.

Clara could never eat alone, except at home in the context of compulsive rituals. In the 3 years at a local commuting college (following her acute breakdown at an out-of-town school), she came home daily for lunch, never once entering the college cafeteria. Clara could eat out with her family or boyfriends (regarded as "meal tickets"). They had to help overcome her painful indecision with the expensive menu. Whenever she violated a food ritual, Clara was gripped in the almost delusional conviction of instantaneous obesity; days passed before she summoned the courage to weigh herself. But first she had to use a laxative and a depilatory, to shave down the ounces.

Clara regarded food as a kind of poison. The compulsive rituals which protected her against the poison were subjectively experienced as external controls, substituting for the controlling symbiotic object. Drugs were regarded similarly, as poisons which would erode her controls. Alcohol was excepted; Clara considered liquor not as a drug-poison, but as a ritual relaxant potion (two drinks on an empty stomach) to overcome strong inhibitions in heterosexual relationships.

Unlike the situation with Mrs. Y, who was consistently fearful and placatingly indulgent of Sally, the control would shift back and forth between Clara and her mother in their symbiotic dyad. This exchange of roles between mother and child was the prototype of Clara's two kinds of heterosexual relationships: controlling and cruel with the nice, passive men; submissive and masochistic with the dominating, cruel ones.

Sally used her "downs," including heroin, with a sense of domination deriving from that exerted over her parents, to reinforce a regressive narcissistic withdrawal from real objects into a state of self-sufficient omnipotence. Peer relations were based primarily on the shared interest in the drug. Clara, somewhat more advanced in separation-individuation, felt herself separate and weak and yearned for a symbiotic relationship. After years of superficial heterosexual promiscuity combined with conscious homosexual attraction to her mother's most feminine friends, Clara fell in love with a girl her own age. In this lesbian relationship, the love object represented a fusion of the idealized self and the idealized mother. Clara's strong masculine identifications, to the fore in her active courting, receded in the actual lovemaking, in which the yearned-for symbiotic merger was enacted.

Both patients have exquisitely vulnerable narcissistic self-esteem regulation, subject to abrupt deflation into the abyss of utter worthlessness. Both scramble frenetically for external supplies to restore self-esteem by recapturing the sense of omnipotence. They turn to different sources, however. Sally's source is heroin, while Clara obtains narcissistic supplies from a variety of object relationships. The therapeutic prerequisite with Sally is to block her reliance on heroin, leaving no choice but the substitution of proferred object relationships. This, in effect, forces her into a predicament comparable to Clara's. Only then can the pathological immaturities be confronted.

DISCUSSION OF TREATMENT

A modification of psychoanalytic psychotherapy suitable for borderline patients described by Kernberg (1968) includes systematic analysis of the negative transference in the here-and-now, and promotion of the observing function of the ego in a structured therapeutic situation which sets limits and blocks acting out of the transference. The limits imposed include the suppression of drug taking.

These represent the basic conditions promoting change and growth in therapy. Classical analysis unmodified provokes regression and acting out which is either too gratifying or disorganizing to be utilizable in treatment. By contrast, the excessively rigid and controlled structure of some mass treatment programs may send the negative transference underground. Suppression of the symptom in such a setting may derive from identification with the aggressor in the form of a personified introject; or it may be an outward compliance without genuine change. In either case, the potential for relapse is obvious.

Sally has a long way to go in her treatment, but significant advances have been made in fashioning conditions favoring an eventual positive outcome. Her parents continue active participation in therapy so that paternal denial and maternal fearfulness no longer provide oral gratification without limit setting. Hitherto, Sally could conceal, from herself and others, her profound dependency on her parents by her ability to obtain their gratification of her dependent needs and by the ease with which she shifted from one superficial need-satisfying object relationship with boyfriends to another. Sally's drug use cannot be considered satisfactorily suppressed, despite the utilization of professionally trained companions, so that the more strictly supervised setting of a drug treatment center or psychiatric hospital will be required before she can come to grips with the issues Kernberg stresses.

In conclusion, heroin abuse is symptomatic behavior. Nomothetic generalization about "the heroin addict" presses a false facade of uniformity upon a population heterogeneous in type of use, etiology, personality organization, amenability to different forms of psychotherapeutic intervention and prognosis. This presentation has focused upon the subgroup of borderline personalities who employ heroin in Type III use. The rational approach to a specific prescription of therapy in heroin use is through the careful metaphychological diagnosis of the personality of the heroin user. The patient is more than a heroin user; he is an individual with his own particular constellation of psychopathology which includes taking heroin.

REFERENCES

Deutsch, H. Some forms of emotional disturbance and their relationship to schizophrenia. *Psychoanal Q*, 11:301-321, 1942.

Freud, S. *On Narcissism.* (1914) SE 14:67-102. London: Hogarth Press, 1957a.

──────. *Mourning and Melancholia.* (1917) SE 14:243-258. London: Hogarth Press, 1957b.

Grinker, R.R., Sr., Werble, B., and Drye, R.C. *The Borderline Syndrome.* New York: Basic Books, 1968.

Hoch, P., and Polatin, P. Pseudoneurotic forms of schizophrenia. *Psychiatric Q*, 23:248-276, 1949.

Kernberg, O. The treatment of patients with borderline personality organization. *Int J Psychoanal*, 40:600-619, 1968.

Knight, R.P. Borderline states. *Bull. Menninger Clinic*, 17:1-12, 1953.

Loewenstein, R.M., Newman, L., Schur, M., and Solnit, A.J., eds. *Psychoanalysis—A General Psychology.* New York: Int. Univ. Press, 1966.

Minuchin, S., Montalvo, B., Guervey, B.C., Jr., Rosman, B.L., and Schumer, T. *Families of the Slums, An Exploration of their Structure and Treatment.* New York: Basic Books, 1967.

Pavenstedt, E. *The Drifters: Children of Disorganized Lower Class Families.* Boston: Little, Brown, 1967.

Pfeiffer, E. *Disordered Behavior: Basic Concepts in Clinical Psychiatry.* New York: Oxford Univ. Press, 1975.

Schmideberg, M. The borderline patient. In: *American Handbook of Psychiatry,* S. Arieti, ed., 1:398-418. New York: Basic Books, 1959.

Stoller, R.J. *Splitting: A Case of Female Masculinity.* New York: Quadrangle-N.Y. Times Book Co., 1973.

Wieder, H., Kaplan, E.H., Drug use in adolescents: Psychodynamic meaning and pharmacogenic effect. *Psychoanal Study Child,* 24:399-431, 1969.

Yorke, C. A critical review of some psychoanalytic literature on drug addiction. *Br J Med Psychol,* 43:141-159, 1970.

CHAPTER 10

Ego Functions in Drug Users

William A. Frosch, M.D., and Harvey Milkman, Ph.D.

Multidrug experimentation, particularly by adolescents, and polydrug abuse have recently become foci of professional attention, at times to the exclusion of investigating preferential drug use and abuse. Although it is clear that many users go through a period of testing and trying, at least some settle on a specific preferred drug. This choosing, clearly in part socially determined (e.g., by availability, peer approval, etc.), must also tell us something of importance concerning personality and perhaps physiologic variables determining drug choice, abuse, and maintenance in the drug subculture.

These considerations led us to select a group of drug abusers with strong stated preference for either heroin or amphetamine and to examine selected aspects of personality structure under both abstinent and preferred intoxicated conditions. Using Bellak and Hurvich's (1969) Interview and Rating Scale for Ego Functioning, "preferential" users of heroin (N=10) or amphetamines (N=10) were interviewed under conditions of abstinence and intoxication with their respectively chosen drug. Normals (N=10) were interviewed twice while abstinent. Data were analyzed, qualitatively and quantitatively, to answer: a) how do preferential users differ from normals and each other under abstinent conditions, b) how do they differ under conditions of intoxication, c) how does the drug user differ within himself under conditions of abstinence and intoxication?

Kramer's (1967) notion of preferential use was applied and supported. In a sample of more than 30 drug admissions to Bellevue Psychiatric Hospital, more than 75 percent stated a specific preference for either heroin or amphetamine. All subjects had experienced both drugs, but the majority stated a strong preference and prolonged involvement with either heroin or amphetamine. The criteria for drug dependence were intravenous administration and minimal levels of use in the past month (amphetamines, more than nine times; heroin, more than five times). Subjects were white, male, middle class, 20-30 years of age, and nonpsychotic. Each heroin user was interviewed while abstinent and under the influence of 15 mg. morphine, given intramuscularly, in a clinical setting. Amphetamine users were interviewed while abstinent and intoxicated with 30 mg. (oral) dextroamphetamine sulfate, also in a clinical setting. Normals were used as a control and interviewed twice while abstinent. Abstinence was determined by self-report and urine analysis. Interviews were spaced 1 to 2 weeks apart, taped, and the interviewer was blind to subject types and conditions of intoxication. The results pertain to a specific type of drug-using population (white, middle class) but may also be applicable to minority groups.

Initial impressions suggested distinct relationships between personality style and drug preference (Milkman and Frosch 1973). The amphetamine abuser coped with his difficulties with an inflated sense of self-worth and active confrontation with his environment. The heroin abuser was consciously depressed and despairing, and withdrew from an environment perceived as hostile and threatening.

Each subject participated in two semistructured interviews and was rated in accord with Bellak and Hurvich's (1969) Interview and Rating Scale for Ego Functioning. Scoring yields a composite quantitative index of "general adaptive strength," as well as specific scores for degree of impairment in each of 11 specified ego functions: 1) Autonomous Functioning, 2) Synthetic-Integrative Functioning, 3) Sense of Competence, 4) Reality Testing, 5) Judgment, 6) Sense of Reality, 7) Regulation and Control of Drives, Affects and Impulses, 8) Object Relations, 9) Thought Processes, 10) Defensive Functioning, and 11) Stimulus Barrier. The scale also provides measures for Libidinal and Aggressive Drive strengths. (See figures 1, 2, and 3. Because Stimulus Barrier ratings are qualitative, i.e., high, medium, or low, rather than quantitative, this variable is omitted from the figures.) Ratings are calculated on a 13-point system with each ego function subscale (e.g., reality testing) constructed such that a low rating indicates maladaptive functioning, and a score of 9 or higher indicates the normal range. Scales for drive strengths differ in that a middle score of 7 is considered adaptive while low scores reflect excessive drive strength and high scores reflect insufficient drive strengths.

The test data were submitted to analyses of variances for comparison of heroin and amphetamine users, under abstinent and intoxicated conditions, with a control group of unintoxicated

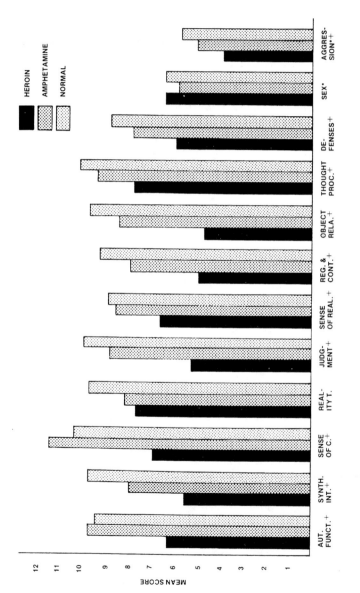

Fig. 1. Mean ego function ratings for amphetamine S's, heroin S's, and normals in the abstinent condition with ratings for libidinal and aggressive drive strengths.

* High score reflects lower strength drive.   + p < .05 (amphetamine vs. heroin)

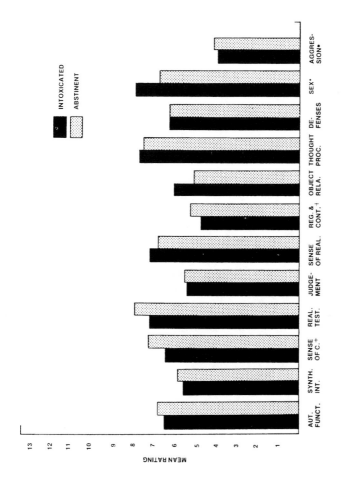

Fig. 2. Mean ego function ratings for heroin users in abstinent and intoxicated conditions with scores for libidinal and aggressive drive strength. (N = 10)

* High score reflects low drive strength.   + p ⟨ .05

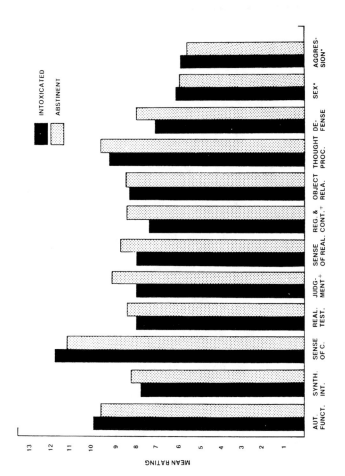

Fig. 3. Mean ego function ratings for amphetamine users in abstinent and intoxicated conditions with scores for libidinal and aggressive drive strength. (N = 10)

* High score reflects low drive strength.   + p < .05

normals. Under the abstinent condition, both drug-using populations showed subnormal ego function ratings in most categories. With the exception of Reality Testing, amphetamine users exhibited significantly higher ego strength than heroin users, whether or not they were intoxicated. There were no statistically significant differences between normal and amphetamine users, and Libidinal Drive Strength did not show significance under any of the comparisons made. In most cases ego functioning was lower in the intoxicated condition with significant differences observed for three variables.

Although relative to heroin users, ego functioning is more adaptive in amphetamine users when both groups are in the intoxicated condition, one cannot, unequivocally, extend this finding outside of the laboratory situation. Experimental doses of 30 mg. and 15 mg. for amphetamine and heroin users, respectively, may not be comparable in effect to average "field" doses of 310 mg. and 100 mg. Even at our reduced dose range, however, the results suggest a trend, in both groups, for ego functioning to be negatively affected by the utilization of their respective drugs. Six of the 10 means observed-for-heroin users are lower in the intoxicated condition. Eight of the 10 means observed-for-amphetamine users are lower in the intoxicated condition. There are four cases in which ego functioning is significantly lower in the intoxicated condition: Regulation and Control of Drive, Affect and Impulse (for both groups), Judgment (for amphetamine users), Sense of Competence (for heroin users). A nearly significant result is observed for Reality Testing (this function is lower for both groups in the intoxicated condition). It is expected that under conditions of higher doses, greater impairment of ego functioning may be observed and more significance obtained.

For the purposes of this presentation, we will only discuss a selection of the measured individual ego functions. The full data will be available elsewhere (Milkman and Frosch, in press).

Autonomous Functioning is assessed according to the degree of impairment of apparatuses of primary autonomy (functional disturbances of sight, hearing, intention, language, memory, learning or motor function) and secondary autonomy (disturbances in habit patterns, learned complex skills, work routines, hobbies and interests). While amphetamine users are relatively unimpaired in this area, heroin users are subject to moderately high interference, by conflict, of their apparatuses of primary and secondary autonomy. Interview material revealed specific problems in concentration with difficulty carrying out routine tasks and skilled behaviors.

Sense of Competence is based on the subject's overt, conscious statement of his feelings of adequacy. No attempt was made at assessing the underlying dynamics for this statement (e.g., unconscious denial of helplessness, etc.). Scores reflect the person's expectation of success or the subjective experience of actual performance (how he feels about how he does and what he can do). Amphetamine users have a significantly higher Sense of Competence across both interview conditions. Although there is no significant drug effect for amphetamine users on this variable, the obtained mean is higher in the intoxicated condition. While amphetamine appears to bolster feelings of adequacy, heroin seems to have the opposite effect. The amphetamine user denies feelings of helplessness and inadequacy; the heroin user is prone to accept feelings of hopelessness and despair. These findings are consistent with clinical impressions that the amphetamine user is grandiose and the heroin user is concerned with survival and self-maintenance.

Judgment evaluates the subject's anticipation of the consequences of intended behaviors (legal culpabilities and social censure, disapproval or inappropriateness) and the extent to which manifest behavior reflects the awareness of these consequences. Amphetamine users show significantly more adaptive Judgment than heroin users across both interview conditions. Although drug intoxication does not significantly impair the Judgment of heroin users in this situation, amphetamine users show a significant decrement in their judgmental capacity while under the influence of amphetamine. The heroin user's Judgment is so defective that he repeatedly encounters danger in health, work and interpersonal relationships. Although he may verbally anticipate the consequences of his actions, manifest behavior rarely reflects this awareness. For the amphetamine user, poor Judgment usually occurs in fairly encapsulated or conflict-related areas.

Sense of Reality rates the extent to which external events are experienced as real and as being embedded in a familiar context; the extent to which the body and its functioning are experienced as familiar and unobtrusive; the degree to which the person has developed individuality and self-esteem. The data show significant differences between heroin and amphetamine users across both interview conditions. The heroin user appears as an individual of quasi-stable sense of identity dependent on outside sources. When external signals and cues are absent, identity can become poorly integrated. Occasional derealization and depersonalization are observed with some unrealistic feelings about the body. In most cases self-esteem is low. The amphetamine user is less dependent on environmental feedback, and depersonalization-like phenomena are more likely to occur under unusual conditions (falling asleep, drugs, radical environmental changes). The heroin user's need for external regulation of self-esteem is seen as a potent factor in the relative success of the therapeutic community. Peer pressure is generated to support nonaddictive behavior. For an individual lacking in a sense of independent identity, the group ideal is easily adopted and until the user returns to his former community, his drug taking and criminal activity may be curtailed.

Regulation and Control of Drive, Affects and Impulses refers to the directness of impulse expression and the effectiveness of delay and control mechanisms; the degree of frustration tolerance and the extent to which drive derivatives are channeled through ideation, affective expression and manifest behavior. Amphetamine users are significantly higher than heroin users under intoxicated and abstinent conditions. Both groups display significantly less Regulation and Control of Drive, Affects and Impulses in the intoxicated condition. The significant drug effect for this function is particularly interesting because it suggests that under intoxication both groups might be expected to have less impulse control and present a greater danger to themselves and/or the community. The heroin user appears as an individual given to sporadic rages, tantrums or binges. Periods of overcontrol may alternate with flurries of impulsive breakthroughs. This may be observed dramatically when the user voluntarily submits himself to extended periods of increased environmental structure, in drug programs, where impulse expression is minimized. Temporarily the user appears to have adequate impulse control. Suddenly and without warning, however, impulses gain the upper hand and the user is seen on a self-destructive binge. Disciplinary action is taken and once again impulses are quieted through self-regulation, authoritative, and peer pressures. The cycle tends to repeat.

For the amphetamine user, impulse expression is less direct, pervasive and frequent. Aggressive behavior is more often verbal than physical and fantasies predominate over unusual behavior. Manifestations of drive-related fantasies are seen in quasi-artistic productions such as "speed freak" drawings where primitive and threatening fantasies are portrayed through massive expenditures of compulsive energy. The amphetamine user may sit for hours drawing frightened faces, decapitated bodies, etc.

Object Relations takes into account the degree and kind of relatedness to others; the extent to which present relationships are adaptively patterned upon older ones; the extent of object constancy. Amphetamine users are significantly more effective in Object Relations than heroin users, across abstinent and intoxicated conditions. It is interesting to note that for heroin users, the obtained mean for this function is higher in the intoxicated condition.

Perhaps in this dose range, heroin tends to reduce anxiety and allows for a smoother and more relaxed communication between people. This notion supports Hartmann's (1969) observation that "there is an attempt to overcome the lack of affectionate and meaningful object relations through the pseudo-fusion with other drug takers during their common experience." The heroin user is generally detached from people while under stress, and strives for nurturant relationships, of a dependent nature, leading to stormy or strained attachments. The amphetamine user, although more successful in Object Relations, tends to become involved in relationships with strong, unresolved Oedipal elements. Castration concerns tend to manifest themselves in unusual and extreme sexual behaviors, such as Don Juanism and homosexuality. Underlying concerns about masculinity and adequacy are expressed through compulsive sexual activity and a boasting attitude of sexual prowess and potency. Relationships may, however, endure for long periods of time, although they rarely have the stability and sustaining power of the idealized marital situation.

Stimulus Barrier indicates the subject's threshold for, sensitivity to, or awareness of stimuli impinging upon various sensory modalities; the nature of responses to various levels of sensory stimulation in terms of the extent of disorganization, withdrawal or active coping mechanisms employed to deal with medium or low Stimulus Barriers. Amphetamine users have significantly higher Stimulus Barriers than heroin users in the abstinent condition. Examination of the raw data revealed that 6 of 10 amphetamine users interviewed were rated high on this variable and 9 of 10 heroin users were rated low. The data tend to support Ellinwood's (1967) suggestions concerning biological predilections for certain drugs. Although it may be argued that long-term involvement with particular drugs may have specific effects on stimulus thresholds, Stimulus Barrier is considered to be the most constitutionally based ego function (Bellak and Hurvich 1969). The data suggest that amphetamine users, with biologically high thresholds for excitatory stimulation, are seeking homeostasis through self-medication. Amphetamine seems to put the user into closer touch with environmental stimuli which might otherwise be unavailable because of constitutionally based high Stimulus Barriers. Conversely, the heroin user may have a predisposition toward excessive vulnerability to environmental stimuli. He seeks to raise stimulus thresholds, allowing more adaptive function in a world of relatively painful and extreme stimulation.

Aggressive Drive Strength assesses: overt aggressive behavior (frequency and intensity); associated and substitute aggressive behavior (verbal expressions, etc.); fantasies and other ideation; dreams; symptoms, defenses and controls. Heroin users have significantly higher Aggressive Drive Strength than amphetamine users across both interview conditions. There is no apparent difference between normals and amphetamine users on this variable. The heroin user is seen as an individual whose overt acts of aggression are considerably more intense and frequent than average. The presence of physical assaultiveness and multiple suicide gestures is common. Hostile punning and witty repartee are often observed. It is speculated that the relative success of residential treatment programs is related to this phenomenon. Intensive confrontation in group therapy (a major treatment modality in drug programs) provides an outlet for excessive aggressive energy. Violent verbal expressions are often encouraged and readily tolerated, thus reducing the user's tendencies toward repression and withdrawal. This approach seems to be effective in decreasing the heroin user's potential for overt violence of an inner and outer directed nature. For the amphetamine user, aggressive energy appears to be less excessive and is channeled more adaptively. Periodic breakthroughs of violence occur, but, with the exception of amphetamine psychosis, these expressions are usually not as frequent or intense as the heroin user's. Fantasies of violence are usually expressed verbally and sometimes find their expression through identification with radical political groups. This finding, greater hostility in heroin addicts than amphetamine abusers, is echoed in a recent study (Gossop and Roy 1976) using different scales and a different population.

DISCUSSION

Although the observations for this study were made while male users were under abstinent and somewhat intoxicated conditions, it must be recalled that our subjects had all been heavy drug users for several years. It is, therefore, difficult to know if our findings represent a factor in the etiology of the pattern of drug use or the result of such drug use and its imposed life patterns. However, quantitative analyses and clinical impressions provide a framework for conceptualizing possible psychological differences between preferential users of heroin and amphetamine. Some speculate that these differences are related to early, pre-drug patterns of childhood experiences.

Having once experienced a particular drug-induced pattern of ego functioning, the user may seek it out again for defensive purposes as a solution to conflict or for primary delight. This seeking out of a special ego state will be related to the individual's previous needs for the resolution of conflict or anxiety. If a particular drug-induced ego state resolves a particular conflict, an individual may seek out that particular drug when in that conflict situation. This will result in preferential choice of drug.

Wieder and Kaplan (1969) define the altered ego state induced by opiates as "blissful satiation." As Savitt (1963) points out, the elation produced by these drugs has been stressed out of proportion to the sleep or stupor which follows. The transient euphoria preceding the stupor may be related both to the decreased pressure of the drives, libidinal and aggressive, and to the sense of gratification of needs. The user "seeks desperately to fall asleep as a surcease from anxiety and the drug provides obliteration of consciousness. Well expressed in the vernacular, the addict 'goes on the nod.' "

The heroin user, who characteristically maintains a tenuous equilibrium via withdrawal and repression, bolsters these defenses by pharmacologically inducing a state of decreased motor activity, under-responsiveness to external situations and reduction of perceptual intake: ". . . [a] state of quiet lethargy . . . [is] . . . conducive to hypercathecting fantasies of omnipotence, magical wish fulfillment, and self-sufficiency. A most dramatic effect of drive dampening experienced subjectively as satiation may be observed in the loss of libido and aggression and the appetites they serve" (DeQuincey 1907, p. 79).

Though, as expected, the dramatic effects outlined above were not brought on by our low level, experimental dose, the observed data points in a parallel direction. Elevated scores for Object Relations, and Sense of Reality, suggest greater relaxation and less pressure from the drives. Though not significantly lower, the mean score for Libidinal Drive Strength points to a dampening of sexual appetite. Wieder and Kaplan further point out that this style of coping is reminiscent of the Narcissistic Regressive Phenomenon described by Mahler (1967), as an adaptive pattern of the second half of the first year of life. It occurs after the specific tie to the mother has been established and is an attempt to cope with the disorganizing quality of even her brief absences. It is as if the child must shut out affective and perceptual claims from other sources during the mother's absence. This formulation is consistent with earlier remarks by Fenichel (1945). Addicts are "fixated to a passive-narcissistic aim" where objects are need-fulfilling sources of supply. The oral zone and skin are primary, and self-esteem is dependent on supplies of food and warmth. The drug represents these supplies. Addicts are intolerant of tension and cannot stand pain or frustration. In our study, the notion of low pain thresholds is supported by the observation that 9 of the 10 heroin users interviewed received a "low" rating for Stimulus Barrier. Drug effects alleviate these difficulties by reproducing the "earliest narcissistic state." The specific need gratification of the passive-narcissistic regression reinforces drug-taking behavior.

The overall decrement in ego functioning (which is clearly observed in our study, even at this low dose) and the pressures of physiological dependency, however, set the groundwork for a vicious cycle. The heroin user must increasingly rely on a relatively intact ego to procure drugs and attain satiation. Ultimately he is driven to withdrawal from heroin by the discrepancy between intrapsychic needs and external demands. Hospitalization, incarceration or self-imposed abstinence subserve the user's need to resolve his growing conflicts with reality.

In contrast to heroin and other sedative drugs, amphetamines have the general effect of increasing functional activity. Extended wakefulness, alleviation of fatigue, insomnia, loquacity and hypomania are among the symptoms observed. Subjectively there is an increase in awareness of drive feelings and impulse strength as well as heightened feelings of self-assertiveness, self-esteem and frustration tolerance. Though not statistically significant, our observations support most of these generalizations. Amphetamine intoxication produced in our subjects elevated scores on Autonomous Functioning and Sense of Competence. Interview material suggests a feeling of heightened perceptual and motor abilities accompanied by a stronger sense of potency and self-regard.

As in the case of heroin, the alterations induced by amphetamine intoxication are syntonic with the user's characteristic modes of adaptation. This formulation is in agreement with the observations of Angrist and Gershon (1969) in their study of the effects of large doses (up to 50 mg./hour) of amphetamine: ". . . it appears that in any one individual, the behavioral effects tend to be rather consistent and predictable. . . . Moreover these symptoms tended to be consistent with each person's personality and 'style.'"

Energizing effects of amphetamine serve the user's needs to feel active and potent in the face of an environment perceived as hostile and threatening. Massive expenditures of psychic and physical energy are geared to defend against underlying fears of passivity. Wieder and Kaplan (1969) suggest that the earliest precursor to the amphetamine user's mode of adaptation is the "practicing period" described by Mahler (1967). This period "culminates around the middle of the second year in the freely walking toddler seeming to feel at the height of his mood of elation. He appears to be at the peak of his belief in his own magical omnipotence which is still to a considerable extent derived from his sense of sharing in his mother's magic powers." There is an investment of cathexis in "the autonomous apparatuses of the self and the functions of the ego; locomotion, perception, learning."

Our subject's inflated self-value and emphasis on perceptual acuity and physical activity support the notion that amphetamine use is related to specific premorbid patterns of adaptation. The consistent finding that ego structures are more adaptive in the amphetamine user than they are in the heroin user suggests that regression is to a later phase of psychosexual development.

Reich's (1960) comments on the "etiology of compensatory narcissistic inflation" may provide further insight into the personality structure of amphetamine users. "The need for narcissistic inflation arises from a striving to overcome threats to one's bodily intactness." Under conditions of too frequently repeated early traumatizations, the primitive ego defends itself via magical denial. "It is not so, I am not helpless, bleeding, destroyed. On the contrary, I am bigger and better than anyone else." Psychic interest is focused "on a compensatory narcissistic fantasy whose grandiose character affirms the denial." The high level artistic and political aspirations witnessed in our subjects appear to be later developmental derivatives of such infantile fantasies of omnipotence. Although the amphetamine user subjectively experiences increments in functional capacity and self-esteem, biological and psychological systems are ultimately drained of their resources. As in the case of heroin, our study points to an overall decrement in ego functioning under the influence of amphetamine. The recurrent disintegration of mental and physical functioning is a dramatic manifestation of the amphetamine syndrome.

Recent workers (Hekimian and Gershon 1968) have typically focused on the seemingly indiscriminate use of a variety of psychotropic agents. Multiple drug abuse or "status-medicamentosus" (Wahl 1967) has been well documented. By viewing the problem from the perspective of preferred drug used, we have defined differences between users, but note many basic similarities. An underlying sense of low self-esteem is defended against by the introduction of a chemically induced altered state of consciousness. The drug state helps to ward off feelings of helplessness in the face of a threatening environment. Pharmacological effect reinforces characteristic defenses deployed to reduce anxiety. Drugged consciousness appears to be a regressive state which is reminiscent of, and may recapture, specific phases of early child development.

The continuing controversy over how to treat whom among drug users is evidence of our lack of understanding of factors which act to maintain drug users in the drug world. We know relatively little about the inner needs and wishes of drug users or about the details of the ways drug use satisfies those needs and wishes. Differences in personality structure and function, such as those we describe in preferential users of heroin and amphetamine, may provide clues which would permit careful delineation of a variety of treatment programs designed to meet the needs of a particular group of drug users. Prediction of the appropriateness of a particular user to a specific treatment program would increase the likelihood of the user remaining in treatment and increase the likelihood of successful outcome. Choosing the right drug in treating infection or psychosis is recognized as important, often crucial; we suggest a likely parallel in the treatment of drug use.

A successful treatment program must provide the user with alternative modes of satisfying those inner needs and wishes previously resolved through drug use. Such alternative modes may include new patterns of discharge, gratification, or defense. The design of such programs requires more detailed knowledge than is currently available. Most workers have tended to lump together, rather than to distinguish between, forms of drug use. In addition to such variables as the ego functions reported here, studies of cognitive style and of physiologic responsiveness are likely to prove important.

REFERENCES

Angrist, B., and Gershon, S. Amphetamine abuse in New York City, 1966-1968. *Semin Psychiat*, 1:195-207, 1969.

Bellak, L., and Hurvich, M. A systematic study of ego functions. *J Nerv Ment Dis*, 148:569-585, 1969.

DeQuincey, T. *Confessions of an English Opium-Eater*. New York: E.P. Dutton, 1907. p. 79.

Ellinwood, E.H. Amphetamine psychosis: I. Description of the individuals and process. *J Nerv Ment Dis*, 144:273-283, 1967.

Fenichel, O. *The Psychoanalytic Theory of Neurosis*. New York: Norton, 1945.

Gossop, M.R., and Roy, A. Hostility in drug dependent individuals: Its relation to specific drugs, and oral or intravenous use. *Br J Psychiatry*, 128:188-193, 1976.

Hartmann, D. A study of drug-taking adolescents. *Psychoanal Study Child*, 24:384-397, 1969.

Hekimian, L.J., and Gershon, S. Characteristics of drug abusers admitted to a psychiatric hospital. *JAMA*, 205:125-130, 1968.

Kramer, J.C., Fischman, V.S., and Littlefield, D.C. Amphetamine abuses. Patterns and effects of high doses taken intravenously. *JAMA*, 201:305-309, 1967.

Mahler, M. On human symbiosis and the vicissitudes of individuation. *J Am Psychoanal Assoc*, 15:740-760, 1967.

Milkman, H. and Frosch, W.A. On the preferential abuse of heroin and amphetamine. *J Nerv Ment Dis*, 156:242-248, 1973.

_____. The Drug of Choice. *J Psychedelic Drugs*, Vol. 9, Issue 1, in press.

Reich, A. Pathologic forms of self-esteem regulation. *Psychoanal Study Child*, 15:215-232, 1960.

Savitt, R.A. Psychoanalytic studies on addiction and ego structure in narcotic addiction. *Psychoanal Q*, 32:43-57, 1963.

Wahl, C.W. Diagnosis and treatment of status medicamentosis. *Dis Nerv Syst*, 28:318-322, 1967.

Wieder, H. and Kaplan, E.H. Drug use in adolescents. Psychodynamic meaning and pharmacogenic effect. *Psychoanal Study Child*, 24:399-431, 1969.

CHAPTER 11

Psychiatric Aspects of Opiate Dependence: Diagnostic and Therapeutic Research Issues

George E. Woody, M.D.

INTRODUCTION

This paper reports on the second in a series of meetings on the psychodynamics and psychotherapy of addiction (see Chapter 1). These meetings represent a reawakening of interest in the psychological makup of addicts and in the perspective that psychoanalysis can contribute to understanding and treating them. Addicts have many different personality structures, and analysis, because it is a special and unique way of getting information about personality, may be able to add something to our understanding of addiction. One might hope to develop a psychology of addiction based on analytic insights. A possible result may be that certain abuse patterns or personality types can be identified which will lead to modifications in treatment approaches. In addition, a subgroup of addicts may be identified that will benefit from psychoanalytically oriented psychotherapy.

This was a two-day meeting and contained both formal presentations and informal give-and-take discussions among all members, addressing seven major areas:

- A review of the first meeting
- Priorities of this meeting
- Problem areas to consider in designing research involving narcotic addicts
- Factors to be measured in psychodynamic-psychotherapy studies with addicts

- A proposed design for evaluating psychotherapy in drug abuse treatment
- Other proposed studies
- Summary—future directions

This paper is a composite of contributions made by all participants and is designed to be understandable and interesting to readers from analytic and nonanalytic backgrounds. Definitions of analytic terms are included in the Appendix. The terms selected include the major ones used in the meetings and are taken from *A Glossary of Psychoanalytic Terms and Concepts*, edited by Burness E. Moore, M.D., and Bernard D. Fine, M.D., published by the American Psychoanalytic Association, second edition, 1968. The discussions were often wide ranging, employing concepts from general psychiatry and addiction research as well as psychoanalysis. Two main themes emerged from group discussions: (1) *analytic ideas* relating to the understanding and treatment of addiction and (2) *research designs* that can be developed to test these ideas. These themes are common threads that run through each section of this paper.

REVIEW OF THE INITIAL MEETING

The purpose of the first meeting, held on April 2 and 3, 1976, was to reexamine analytic theory for its relevance to understanding opiate addiction. It was the beginning of an attempt to develop practical applications of analytic ideas in the field of drug addiction. Participants shared a conviction that addiction needs a depth psychology and that analytic theory can be a useful tool in its development. Drs. Khantzian and Treece reviewed the discussion and papers presented at this meeting (see Chapter 2). A summary follows.

The early analytic views of addiction were based on libido theory. They held that addiction resulted from libidinal fixation (notably oral), with regression to that state of psychic development. The need to explain the relationship between drug abuse, defenses, impulse control, affective disturbances, and adaptive mechanisms led to the recent shift emphasizing ego psychology.

Participants agreed that serious ego pathology was often associated with drug abuse and most felt that this is indicative of profound developmental disturbances. Problems in the relationship between the ego and affects emerged as a key area of difficulty, including affective experiencing, control, intensity, and ambivalence.

The group members agreed that multi-modality treatment and pluralism were sensible approaches to therapy and most felt that psychotherapy can have a positive influence through its ability to correct or improve ego defects. This view is consistent with Kohut's idea that drugs substitute for defects in ego development and that long-term analytically oriented therapy can improve ego functions and thereby reduce or eliminate drug abuse. Comments on the techniques necessary for long-term therapy emphasized the importance of empathy and sensitivity to the addict's fragile self-esteem as well as the importance of walking a thin line between closeness and distance. It was felt that a strictly transference-oriented approach should be modified and that the psychiatrist must play an active role as well as be willing to use psychotropic drugs. Countertransference can be a major pitfall, and one adverse effect of countertransference is that staff members will act out roles that patients unconsciously seek.

In the discussion that followed the presentation of the review, several members commented that analysis can both contribute to and learn from the treatment of addiction. The group expressed an interest in including addictive diseases in the curriculae of analytic institutes, and panel members noted that they knew of only one institute, the Boston Psychoanalytic, that includes courses dealing with addiction.

Two major conclusions resulted from this first meeting:

- That addiction is often associated with *serious ego pathology*
- That *long-term psychotherapy* can reduce this ego pathology and, thereby, lead to a better treatment outcome.

These conclusions are addressed later in this paper and serve as a focus for the research design that resulted from this second meeting.

PRIORITIES OF THE SECOND MEETING

Early in the second meeting, held on March 17 and 18, 1977, the group was asked by Dr. Pollin, Director of NIDA's Division of Research, to examine the ideas presented at the first meeting and to distill and formulate them into testable hypotheses. As a first step he asked the group for ideas that would help decide on the level of approach to this task. Would it be best to focus on the issue of heroin use, heroin abuse, or on some definable behavioral threshold point that is part of an escalating pattern of drug consumption? Or, to look at the problem in another way, to what extent should we focus on heroin use rather than a more general "addictive state"? The recent interest of NIDA to develop studies relating to nicotine abuse was mentioned in this regard. The group was not certain how to answer these questions, and it searched in different directions before reaching a conclusion.

First, several members presented analytic ideas relating to nicotine use. The theoretical contributions of Marcovitz (1969) and Greenacre (1971) on the symbolic meaning of cigarette smoking and inhalation were mentioned. Taking a lead from the issue of nicotine use, studies by Jaffe (1975a) were mentioned that showed similarities between the natural history of cigarette smoking and heroin addiction. Other work by Jaffe (1975b) found evidence that nicotine has the ability to reduce aggressive behavior. Using their own experiences with drug abusers and this material, group members agreed that addictions probably share the following common elements:

- The use of a substance that produces a rapid and pleasurable effect
- Compulsiveness
- Relating to the addictive drug as if it were an object relationship
- Biological changes resulting from drug use
- Cultural and genetic determinants
- Tendencies to be associated with antisocial behavior

Members added that there is a need to examine the factors that *prevent* addiction as well as those that cause it. Several participants commented that studies in this area may be more important than those examining elements that lead to addiction. Studies of the ego processes that operate in addicts, as well as studies that can identify differences between the types of compulsions seen in general psychiatry and those seen in addictions, were mentioned as ways to investigate the personality factors that prevent addiction.

Though each of these areas was relevant to the question asked, none produced a sense that the group had arrived at the area of high priority for which it was looking. Members turned toward the NIDA representatives for their thoughts on priorities. It became clear that NIDA's highest priority has been heroin addiction. This judgment is based on estimates of health and social costs, which indicate that heroin is the most burdensome drug problem from the public health standpoint, followed by amphetamines, barbiturates, hallucinogens, and marihuana, in that order. Alcohol abuse was mentioned as an important area, and NIDA is now working with NIAAA in developing cooperative research projects. Many group members felt that tobacco may be one of the most serious of all addictions from the public health standpoint. There was discussion about controlling tobacco smoking by prohibiting its growth or sale, but it became evident that the complexity of the economic issues involved in tobacco sale and production placed these issues outside the scope of the technical review. The group left open the question of the relative importance of tobacco versus heroin but agreed that heroin addiction is an area of high priority.

The group returned to the conclusion reached at the first meeting —that addiction is often a result of severe ego pathology and that psychotherapy can improve treatment effectiveness. This single issue emerged as the highest priority research area. The group felt that this is a necessary and realistic area to investigate. It is necessary because at this time there is little evidence besides clinical impressions justifying the additional expenses resulting from inclusion of any type of intensive psychotherapy in the routine services provided by narcotic treatment programs. It is realistic because the effectiveness of psychotherapy can be tested using methods that have been developed in other psychotherapy studies.

Other related issues were mentioned such as, if psychotherapy is shown to help, what kind works best? How can addicts be classified? Can psychoanalytic concepts be used to classify them? If classification is possible, can it help guide individuals into a type of therapy that is most likely to give good results? Can the treatment program milieu be modified, based on the psychodynamic understanding of the addict, in order to improve the quality and efficacy of treatment? The group discussed practical benefits that could result from studies that will provide answers. At this point, a priority area had been chosen and the focus of the meeting turned toward issues related to research designs.

PROBLEM AREAS TO CONSIDER IN DESIGNING RESEARCH INVOLVING NARCOTIC ADDICTS

The first research area that the group discussed was the problem of designing studies involving narcotic addicts. Some of these problem areas might be present in any research design, whether it deals with addicts or nonaddicts. Most of the contributions to this part of the discussion were made by members whose experience and training were in research rather than by those experienced in analysis.

Differentiating cause and effect was recognized as, at best, a difficult process. There was discussion about this and questions were raised regarding the pharmacological, cultural, and social impinging variables. Several participants felt that one difficulty in doing research with addicts is in differentiating conditions that existed prior to addiction from those that result from cultural and pharmacological effects acquired in the course of addiction. For example, superego problems could be more a *result of* the laws against heroin use than a *condition* for heroin addiction. Any study of character pathology in addicts will have to deal with this problem. Longitudinal studies were proposed as the best way to separate these variables, but they are expensive and difficult to design and implement. However, it was argued that they would be of great help in separating cause from effect.

An example of cause/effect problems in research is that studies of ego structure in patients being treated with methadone will have to control for any effects produced by methadone itself. It is not known whether methadone changes personality structure, and it was suggested that a nonmethadone treatment group should be used for comparison.

A second area concerned the effects of non-treatment-related life events on therapy outcome. For example, during the course of therapy, a patient may lose or get a job, become engaged or married, move to a different neighborhood, experience the death of a close relative, etc. These events may have a strong influence on outcome, making it difficult to separate therapy effects from the sequelae of life events. Keeping a record of such events that may occur during the course of a study was suggested as a way of allowing them to be taken into consideration when the data are analyzed. Another suggested control for these variables was to do a collaborative study with several clinics. This would increase the number of patients, making it more likely that nontherapeutic interventions would wash out in data analysis.

A third problem was the discontinuous nature of treatment that most addicts experience. A typical addict is not in treatment continuously for longer than a year. Rather, he may be in therapy for 4 months, drop out, return 3 months later and then repeat this pattern. Psychotherapy appointments may be erratic during each treatment cycle. Carefully defining treatment, including length, is one way to control this variable. Contingency payments can be built into the treatment program to encourage patients to participate in their psychotherapy sessions.

A fourth area mentioned was that some patients in drug programs may be brain damaged or have low intelligence. The continuous use of high doses of sedative hypnotics, anoxia resulting from drug overdose, and head injuries suffered in accidents were mentioned as events that produce brain damage in drug addicts. Dr. Wurmser has studied this problem and found that 20 to 30 percent of the patients in his program have minimal brain damage. Others felt that the percentage is less than 20 to 30 percent, but all members agreed that organicity or subnormal intelligence may add special difficulties with psychotherapy studies. The consensus was that such patients should be screened out of research samples. A fifth problem was the possibility of inaccurate conclusions drawn by generalizing from the results of treatment done at only one clinic. Clinics differ in personnel, treatment environment, and policies, and these variables may influence outcome. A treatment that works well at one clinic may not work at another. The group felt that these differences are not easily controlled, but matching clinics in a collaborative study would minimize them. Another member raised the possibility that drug addicts in public treatment programs may not be representative of addicts in general and that the conclusions made from studies involving them may not be generally applicable. The group felt that this problem could be solved if patients from different socioeconomic and ethnic groups were included in the study.

The final area dealt with problems that can result from arriving at estimates of psychopathology by using historical material obtained from patients. Several members had found that the reliability of patient-obtained background information is inversely related to the degree of psychiatric impairment. This will probably lower the reliability of data that can be expected from addicts, because levels of psychopathology are often high among the drug-abusing population. That measures of personality organization may be the most reliable way to evaluate these patients psychiatrically was emphasized by those group members who have had the most analytic experience. The emphasis on measuring personality structure was repeated throughout this meeting and was a major contribution by group members with analytic backgrounds and experience.

ELEMENTS TO MEASURE AND MEASURES TO BE USED IN PSYCHOTHERAPY STUDIES WITH ADDICTS

The second research issue the group addressed was which background and diagnostic factors should be measured and how to measure them. The group arrived at an outline that was a composite of input from members with analytic and general psychiatric perspectives.

All group members felt that *demographic* information such as age, sex, race, occupation, marital status, education, employment, criminal history, intelligence, type of neighborhood, and military history should be included. Intelligence was singled out as especially important and several members indicated that it has been correlated with outcome success in studies of both addicted and nonaddicted psychiatric patients. Dr. Harriet Barr presented results from a study recently completed by her colleague Dr. Arie Cohen (1977) that show what can be done with demographic information. The study included about 1,200 patients who were being treated in a therapeutic community and at methadone programs in the Philadelphia area. Six typologies emerged:

- Type I included individuals who came from very deprived backgrounds. These people had experienced real economic problems. For example, they recalled periods during which they went without essentials such as food or clothing due to lack of money.
- Type II included those distinguished by their criminality, and it included many professional criminals. People in this group were found to use less narcotics than those in the other groups, possibly because they exaggerated their drug problems in order to get favorable treatment within the criminal justice system.
- Type III was a group with a history of problems in the parent-child area. These patients reported parental separations, divorce, missing parents, histories of child abuse, and unhappy childhoods.
- Type IV was a group with a history of psychiatric hospitalization, including suicide attempts.
- Type V consisted of people reporting behavior problems, such as fighting in school, suspension from school, or hyperactivity.
- Type VI was a group who appeared normal and gave no history of problems other than drug abuse.

Analysis of drug-use patterns in these groups showed significant differences, one being that cocaine was used more frequently by the Type II addicts than by other groups.

All members felt that demographic typing such as this is important. The group commented on the importance of including data on patterns of early trauma in demographic information. Dr. Krystal's work on the relationships between trauma, disturbances of affect, and drug abuse was discussed in view of Dr. Barr's report of a group that is distinguished by parental abuse and other evidence of early trauma.

Dr. Kernberg added that the extent of social pressure against a particular drug of abuse is directly related to the severity of the psychopathology of individuals who become addicted to that drug. The group suggested that estimates of *social pressure* should be included in demographic information.

A second area that all members agreed should be included is the patient's *abuse pattern*. The group felt that this is important as a basic piece of information and that it may correlate with other variables such as psychopathology, responses to treatment, age, sex, race, occupation, or education.

A third area was *physiological measures of addiction*. Pupillary dilation, skin temperature, skin resistance, stomach motility, heart rate, respiration, and other psychophysiological indices can be measured and correlated with subjective reports of narcotic withdrawal. Studies using these measures have shown that narcotic withdrawal responses can be conditioned to occur in the presence of various stimuli as well as in response to rapid detoxification or administration of a narcotic antagonist. Addicts have been shown to differ in the ease with which they acquire conditioned withdrawal responses and in the number of stimuli that will produce them. Measures of the intensity of physiological responses to withdrawal and of patients' susceptibility to conditioned withdrawal may serve as indicators of outcome and guides for a treatment approach. For example, someone who is easily conditioned may do better in a program that places emphasis on deconditioning. It may be possible to tailor each patient's therapy to that class of agents that is particularly evocative for him or her. A subsequent reduction in conditioned withdrawal responses may be correlated with treatment effectiveness.

A fourth area involved *therapist variables and the therapeutic process*. The measures of accurate empathy, nonpossessive warmth, and unconditional positive regard developed by Rogers and others may correlate with outcome in addiction treatment (Rogers 1961, Truax 1963, Rogers et al. 1967). Countertransference is also an important variable and two scales were mentioned that can measure it. Therapist charisma is another quality that may relate to outcome. Studies of therapeutic process were also mentioned, as was Luborsky's method that predicts outcome by listening to verbal therapy segments. Videotapes could be made and used to study these things as well as to document the kind of therapy actually being done. But the group felt that therapy process studies should be given a low priority due to the extensive methodological problems that researchers have found in trying to study it.

The fifth area the group felt must be included in any psychiatric study is a *psychiatric diagnostic* study of the patients. This area provoked much discussion because it is complex and involves two general diagnostic levels: (1) the descriptive or general psychiatric and (2) the underlying character or analytic. The descriptive level is the easiest, as the measures suggested here are well known, widely used, and provide a systematic evaluation leading to a psychiatric clinical diagnosis. The group showed a preference for including clinical diagnoses as classified in the American Psychiatric Association's Diagnostic and Statistical Manual (DSM). The group also felt that measures of depression should be included, and the Hamilton and Beck scales were suggested. Other measures discussed were the BPRS (Brief Psychiatric Rating Scale), MMPI (Minnesota Multiphasic Personality Inventory), the Rorschach, and the Psychiatric Diagnostic Criteria developed at Washington University in St. Louis.

Dr. Kernberg suggested that something should be added to these general psychiatric measures that will tap an underlying level of psychopathology, namely, the underlying character structure. This level has been relatively unexplored in addiction research, and it is here that the insights developed through analytic work may be able to broaden our understanding of addiction. He mentioned Luborsky's Health-Sickness Rating scale and Gunderson's scales for differentiating borderlines, psychotics, and neurotics as useful in gaining insights to character structure and function. He also felt that there are three areas of personality organization that are important to measure, and these are:

• The level of defensive functioning
• Identity diffusion
• Reality testing

He has been developing scales to measure these areas. They should be complemented with special tests of personality features. These scales may be of treatment and prognostic relevance. They include quality of object relations as measured by stability, depth (including the ability to fall in love), superego measures, such as the extent of a stable morality; evidence of selfdirected aggression; measures of impulse control and anxiety expression; subliminatory potential; severity of troublesome affects; intelligence; the wish to receive therapy; capacity for meaningful emotional introspection; and likeability. Honesty, as opposed to sociopathy, was emphasized as being of good prognostic value. In the course of the discussion that followed, Weintraub and Aronson's method for measuring defensiveness, Gottchalk's method of using verbal segments to measure anxiety and hostility, and the dependency-counterdependency scale developed by Chodoff and NIMH were referred to and may be useful.

Dr. Treece presented the results of a study she had completed recently in which anxiety and impulsivity were measured in addicts and nonaddicted controls. It involved four groups of subjects who were confined to a women's correctional institution: addicts, controlled nonaddicted users, experimenters, and nonusers. She found that addicts were high on measures of anxiety and impulsivity, whereas experimenters were low on anxiety and low on impulsivity. Controlled users were more anxious than nonusers but were less impulsive. There was a small subgroup of polydrug users who had low anxiety and high impulsivity scores. Nonusers were almost as anxious as addicts, but they differed in having high rather than low field dependency.

Several members commented that the study showed a way in which relationships between anxiety, impulsivity, and cognitive style can be tested experimentally. They felt that this kind of study might serve as a model for using experimental methods to examine relationships between analytic observations, ego functions, and drug abuse.

Dr. Kernberg added that individuals often search for drug effects that are specific to their personality organization. One personality type is found in depressive-masochistic characters who have a sense of destruction or loss of their internal world of object relations. They want to overcome their emptiness with drugs and, at the same time, achieve a sense of euphoria. Drugs for this group represent an infusion of internal goodness, being loved, and loving. This group has the best prognosis. The second personality type consists of those who experience a fragmentation of self, of representations of others, and of affects. These are often schizoid personalities who attempt to use drugs to achieve a sense of organization (to obtain a feeling of "being real" or "being put together again"). The third type, resembling narcissistic personalities, are those who use drugs to replace people or to restore a sense of loss of control over the environment. Drugs permit them a sense of grandiose control of the environment, thereby helping to maintain a sense of superiority. This last group may be very difficult to treat, especially since there is a subgroup with paranoid features.

After pausing and reflecting on the complexity of this entire area, the group concluded that the best approach is a multidimensional one. A study should select the most appropriate and practical measures in each area. Dr. Klerman discussed his positive experiences using this approach in psychotherapy drug studies and pointed out similarities between work done elsewhere and the proposal being discussed here.

Dr. O'Brien and Dr. Pollin suggested that the field would be enhanced by developing a composite instrument that would specifically measure addiction severity. This scale would provide uniformity and standardization in measuring severity of addiction and would be useful in evaluating changes resulting from treatment as well as in comparing patients from different treatment programs.

The focus of the meeting now turned to considerations dealing with a design that can be used for a psychotherapy study.

PROPOSED DESIGN FOR A PSYCHOTHERAPY STUDY

One of the main purposes of the meeting was to formulate research designs and this session dealt with specific proposals. Several were discussed but no single one was selected as the final product. The first step was to determine which treatments should be studied. Three kinds were proposed: supportive, analytic, and a combination of the two. The group agreed that *supportive* therapy should be included. (See Appendix for a definition of "supportive therapy"). Several members focused on problems that can be anticipated in doing *analytic* psychotherapy with addicts. One had to do with addicts' efforts to manipulate therapy to fit their needs for control, support, or gratification. Other problems were the addicts' difficulties in keeping regular appointments, their tendency to externalize problems, and their pattern of dealing with problems in a way that does not reflect high levels of psychological awareness. Using group analytic rather than one-to-one therapy was suggested as a solution, but several members mentioned that they had tried analytically oriented group therapy and experienced attendance problems. Dr. Khantzian recalled that he had solved attendance problems that were occurring in his program by making group therapy mandatory. Other difficulties were mentioned, and the members concluded that group therapy may present too many problems to be used in a psychotherapy study and indicated a preference for one-to-one therapy.

The problems inherent in doing analytic psychotherapy with addicts led to suggestions by several members that the study use a therapy that *combines* supportive and analytic treatments. The group felt that this probably would result in neither good supportive nor good analytic treatment, and they chose to use the purer types. Members suggested that an ongoing monitoring system (videotapes) should be included in the study to provide a means of quality control. This would document what kind of therapy is actually being done. If the therapy is different from that called for in the research design, the tapes will help determine whether this is due to qualities belonging to the therapist or the patient and also will provide a means for maintaining a consistent type of therapy through supervision. There was general agreement that analysis *per se* is impractical, but the possibility of testing it on a selected group was not ruled out.

The second step was to decide if psychotherapy should be tested alone or in combination with methadone. Some members proposed a study that would include patients who are treated with *only* analytic or supportive therapy and *not* with methadone. Several members discussed their negative experiences in trying to treat addicts without methadone and emphasized how they had been impressed by methadone's ability to stabilize addicts and involve them in therapy. The NIDA staff members reminded the group that studies of drug-free therapy are appropriate because the majority of addicts in treatment in the United States are in drug-free modalities. Some discussion followed about the kinds of addicts that can be expected to continue in drug-free treatment, and the group concluded that psychotherapy alone will not keep heroin addicts in outpatient treatment unless special circumstances are operating, such as legal pressures or involvement with a therapeutic community. The members concluded that the value of methadone has been established in outpatient programs and the highest priority of the study is to see if psychotherapy improves methadone treatment.

The value of selecting the best (those patients judged most likely to benefit) and the worst cases versus selection of only the best was discussed. The group felt that much can be learned by studying patients with the worst prognosis, but several members pointed out that including the worst cases may mask positive results and that this could lead to termination of research support for future projects. The group concluded that it is preferable to study the best group first and to include poorer prognosis patients at a later time if positive results are found in the first study. Several members also felt that it is important to design studies with an eye to identifying who needs psychotherapy and who does not. Robins' study of Vietnam veterans was mentioned as having demonstrated that there are many addicts who do not need formal therapy in order to discontinue their addiction to heroin. The group felt that careful diagnosis may be fundamental in deciding on appropriate treatment. For example, analytic psychotherapy may benefit an addict with depression but not one with psychopathy.

These comments led to *one basic design:* randomly assign outpatients to methadone alone, methadone plus analytic therapy, and methadone plus supportive therapy. Variants of this design involved including drug-free groups and/or both good and poor prognosis patients in the random assignment, but this was not preferred.

The group added that it may be more difficult to do this study than it appears. Matching therapists, defining treatment, defining patient groups, guaranteeing quality control, matching clinics, controlling for length of treatment, controlling for life events, and providing large enough numbers of patients are some areas that need clear definition in formulating an experimental design. Three years was estimated as a reasonable duration for the study, and most members felt that a collaborative effort is better than one in which separate studies are done in different clinics. This will allow larger numbers of patients to be studied, thereby providing more control and increasing the significance of the results.

OTHER PROPOSED STUDIES

The discussions also generated ideas for other studies dealing with pharmacology, longitudinal development, therapy variables, and cultural factors related to drug abuse. Several studies were proposed to investigate the *pharmacological* properties of drugs used in treatment. One involved examining the common elements shared by addicting substances and relating them to pharmacological factors of drugs used in treatment. Several group members felt that the rapidly acting drugs are the most useful and singled out the mood-elevating drugs with long latencies for study. Another proposal was to examine whether the slow onset of action of the mood-elevating properties of LAAM is related to difficulties seen in stablizing addicts on this drug.

Issues dealing with *longitudinal developmental processes* generated considerable interest, but the group was aware that they may not be economically feasible. However, leaving economics aside, many possibilities were suggested and they included three areas. First was to design a study that would answer the question, raised in earlier discussions, of whether drug abuse is progressive or regressive. In other words, does it lead to improvement or deterioration of personality function? Stages in the development of drug abuse or identification of drug abuse patterns may be important to identify here, because there may be some patterns that will lead to one result rather than the other. An especially important developmental step is the phenomenon of "losing control." This is a focal point in the progression from drug use to addiction. An extension of earlier studies done by Zinberg (1975) on people who use drugs continuously but irregularly and are not addicted ("chippers") may be able to identify personality elements that act as counterweights against the progression from use to addiction. Measuring ego functions in nonaddicted siblings and further development of the work started by Milkman and Frosch (see Chapter 10) on defensive style and drug of choice may be helpful. The group added that developmental studies involving relationships between personality and addiction would provide a good starting point to verify the observation that the reasons individuals become addicted are often different from those that perpetuate the addiction. Longitudinal studies could also examine the relationship between trauma, affects, impulse control, and drug abuse, a syndrome suggested as commonly associated with the subsequent development of addiction.

A second developmental area is whether aggressive behavior and psychopathy *precede* addiction. A study was mentioned demonstrating that children who have a history of fighting are more likely to become addicts than peers who are more peaceful. Other studies have shown that criminal behavior, as measured by arrest records, precedes heroin addiction. However, the data in these studies are often contaminated, partly because heroin addiction is often the end point in a pattern of polydrug abuse and these drug abuse patterns may contribute to the criminal behavior.

A third area dealt with studies relating to maternal care functions and addiction. It may be possible to identify certain behaviors, attitudes, or interactional patterns that are likely to be associated with the subsequent development of addiction. Children of addicts may have an increased chance of becoming addicted, and physiological changes found to occur in children born to alcoholic mothers may be found in adolescents who become alcoholics. Studies in this area may build on research that is already in progress.

The main proposals dealing with *therapy* were discussed and presented earlier. One further proposal was to try to identify those people for whom total abstinence is appropriate and to determine what differentiates them from those who should be on continuous methadone maintenance.

The last area for study was the *cultural*. The group felt that a study which could identify the social and cultural features that encouraged or discourage drug abuse and addiction will be of great value. Robins' study of Vietnam addicts was mentioned in this regard. Studies of the cultural determinants of use and abuse of diazepam were mentioned as another area of interest, as well as the relationship of psychiatric problems to race. One member's data showed that black addicts have high levels of psychopathology, whereas data presented by others show that it is low. These differences may result from the measures used to determine psychopathology in the studies: APA DSM II criteria were used by some members, and measures of drive states and ego functions were used by others. Further studies in this area are of interest and importance, especially as they may provide data on whether psychopathology necessarily accompanies drug dependence.

SUMMARY—FUTURE DIRECTIONS

Several important conclusions came from this meeting. First, it was agreed that analytic theory has a contribution to make to the understanding of the nature and treatment of drug addiction. The group decided that the highest research priority is a comparative psychotherapy study done on heroin addicts in outpatient methadone treatment. This will include matched patients who are randomly assigned to psychoanalytically oriented, supportive, and no-therapy (methadone only) groups. Poor prognosis patients are to be excluded, as are patients with signs or symptoms of organic brain damage. The study should be a collaborative one and will take about 3 years. Efforts should be made to match the clinics that participate, though this is acknowledged to be difficult.

Measures taken will include the demographic information mentioned earlier and should measure the amount and magnitude of early trauma. Drug abuse patterns should be noted and urine tests results, arrest and employment records are to be recorded at regular intervals. Patients will undergo psychiatric diagnostic studies at intake and throughout the study. They should include general diagnostic tests as well as measures of personality structure appropriate to psychoanalytic classifications of ego pathology. An APA DSM II diagnosis, the Hamilton and Beck measures of depression, and measures of affect expression versus constriction are the preferable general measures. Luborsky's health-sickness rating scale and special tests measuring level of defensive functions, quality of object relations, and accuracy of reality testing are the most important areas of personality function and ego structure.

Physiologic recordings of narcotic withdrawal response to naloxone injections and responses to stimuli that produce conditioned withdrawal responses may also be included. These measures can only be done on a few patients in selected clinics since they are very time consuming and since most clinics do not have the equipment necessary to do them.

Measures of therapist variables, such as those developed by Rogers et al., and countertransference should be included. Therapy sessions should be taped (video or audio) to document the kind of therapy actually being done. Therapeutic process notes or tapes can be included, but, like physiologic measures, studies of therapy process are lengthy and can only be done on a few selected patients.

Another meeting is planned for later this year, and the group consensus was that psychometricians, biostatisticians, and research psychologists should be included, with the aim of further operationalizing clinical concepts and observations into instruments and techniques to be used in experimental studies. Dr. Pollin expressed his strong interest in developing research in this area and his thanks to all the participants.

APPENDIX: DESCRIPTIVE AND THERAPEUTIC TERMS

I. Descriptive Terms

Ego: The ego occupies a position between the primal instincts, based on the physiological needs of the body, and the demands of the outer world. It serves to mediate between the individual and external reality. In so doing, it performs the important function of perceiving the needs of the self, physical and psychic, and the qualities and attitude of the environment. It evaluates, coordinates, and integrates these perceptions so that internal demands can be adjusted to external requirements. In so doing, it sometimes brings relief from drive tensions by a reduction in the intensity of the drives (taming) or by a modification of the external situation. While doing this, it strives to maintain good relations with the external world and with the superego.

Ego Functions: The means used by the ego in performing its duties. These involve:

- *Reality Testing*—This is often distorted in neuroses and is very disturbed in psychoses.
- *Regulation and Control of Drives*—This function is measured by the ability to tolerate anxiety and depression and to delay satisfactions.
- *Object Relations*—This involves the ability to form affectionate, friendly ties to other individuals and to have the ability to maintain them.
- *Thought Processes*—The ability to perceive what is going on and to coordinate, classify, and make sense of perceptions, i.e., to "think."
- *Defensive functions*—Methods used by the ego to protect itself from danger. See "Defenses."
- *Autonomous Functions*—These include perception, motility, intention, intelligence, speech, and language. These are less frequently affected by emotional disturbances than other ego functions.
- *The Synthetic or Organizing Function*—This is the capacity of the ego to unite or organize the drives, tendencies, and functions within the personality in order to enable the person to feel, think, and act in an organized and directed manner.

Defenses: The means available to the ego to protect itself from danger. The integrity of the ego is sometimes threatened by the potential eruption into consciousness of an impulse or wish that has been associated with some real or imagined punishment. This is signaled by feelings of anxiety or guilt that then impel the ego to ward off the wish or drive. Defenses always operate unconsciously so that the person is unaware of what is taking place. The specific methods used are known as defense mechanisms, and these include sublimation, repression, displacement, reaction formation, projection, isolation, and undoing. The operation of such mechanisms may result in a deletion or distortion of some aspect of reality. Being defensive is a general term used to describe a situation in which the ego is struggling to protect itself from danger. Some defenses are indicative of mature ego functioning (sublimation) and others of a more primitive ego (projection).

Ego Defect: Impairment in one or more ego functions.

Superego: The internal representative of the standards of behavior and moral demands imposed from without.

Libido: A concept that refers to a measure of the drive energy of the sexual (pleasurable) instinct, but not denoting sexual appetite or conscious sexual desire. It is one great dynamic force that gives rise to conflict in the course of mental development. The other forces are the self-preservative and aggressive drives. It can be invested in the intrapsychic representation of objects (object libido) or the self (narcissism).

Libido Theory: The theoretical description of a biological maturational sequence of pleasurable phases starting with the oral and ending with the genital phase. The theory assumes that the sources of the sexual instinct are derived from somatic processes that are psychologically experienced as impulses. There are component drives usually associated with specific erogenous zones and wishes or fantasies (a mental organization) representative of each phase. The drive organization is subject to progressions, regressions, and fixation.

Regression: A retreat to an earlier phase of instinctual (libidinal) or mental (ego) organization. Libidinal and ego regression not infrequently occur together. Regression occurs if the individual is presented with difficulties he is unable to master. The extent and form of regression are often determined by unresolved conflicts and anxieties at earlier phases that leave areas of weakness (fixations) to which the individual is likely to regress. For example, at times of stress, a 5-year-old child resumes thumb-sucking (libidinal regression); or, when experiencing difficulty in finding a job, a young man gives up, starts overeating, and wants to be "taken care of" (ego and libidinal regression).

Adaptation: The capacity to cope reasonably yet advantageously with the environment. Successful adaptation provides a gratifying, satisfactory discharge of instinctual forces within the limitations imposed by the external world without pathological alteration of the ego. It requires conforming to reality but does not preclude activity directed toward its change. Adaptation is accomplished by active efforts of the ego, and successful adaptation is regarded as one criterion of healthy ego functioning.

Fixation: The tendency for residuals of earlier libidinal, ego, or superego phases to acquire and retain strong "charges" of psychic energy and to play a significant role in later mental functioning. These then permit the persistence of primitive ways of satisfaction, of relating to people, and of reacting to old dangers.

Narcissism: A concentration of psychological interest upon the self. Normally, an individual's interests are divided between self-concern and concern for the world of things and people around him (object love). Painful self-consciousness and an increased propensity for shame are the outcome of conflicts over narcissism. Exaggerated narcissism may be associated with ego regression and difficulty in object relations.

Object Relations: Personal interactions that include both direct instinctual gratification (sexual, aggressive) as well as instances where gratification is sublimated, as occurs in friendships and in love between parent and child. Primitive object relations are characterized by a relative inability to maintain a love relationship and to accept the limitations and separateness of the loved object. A mixture of love and hate, known as ambivalence, is characteristic of impaired object relationships.

Object Representation: An enduring schema of a particular person modeled by the ego from experiences with that person. Object representation comes to exist independent of real satisfaction. For example, after the object representation of mother is formed, the child perceives her as the same person even when he does not need her to feed or wash him.

Self-Representation: A more enduring schema than the self-image and constructed by the ego out of the multitude of realistic and distorted self-images that the individual has had at different times. It represents the person as he consciously and unconsciously perceives himself. It includes enduring representations of all the experienced body states and all the experienced drives and affects that the individual has consciously or unconsciously perceived in himself at different times in reaction to himself and to the outer world. Together with the object representations, it provides the material for all the ego's adaptive and defensive functions.

Ambivalence: The simultaneous existence of opposite feelings, attitudes, and tendencies directed toward another person, thing, or situation. Ambivalence is universal and not necessarily pathological because there are few affectionate relations that are uncomplicated by hostility, and many hostile relations are tempered by affection. However, when the strength of these conflicting feelings increases to the point where action seems unavoidable yet unccceptable, defensive measures and mental disturbance often result.

II. Therapeutic Terms

Transference: The displacement of patterns of feelings and behavior, originally experienced with significant figures of one's childhood, to individuals in one's current relationships. This process is unconscious and brings about a repetition of attitudes, fantasies, and emotions. The parents are usually the original figures from whom such patterns are displaced, but siblings, grandparents, childhood teachers, and doctors may be contributing figures. Transference may develop in any human relationship. It is of major significance in the analytic process. The demonstration, interpretation, and resolution of transference in the analytic situation constitute the core of analytic therapy. Transference may involve predominately friendly, affectionate, or sexual feelings (positive transference) or mainly aggressive, hostile, or even sadistic wishes (negative transference). A strong working relationship between the patient and therapist is essential to the continuation of analysis, especially during periods of strong negative transference.

Countertransference: Refers to the attitudes and feelings, only partly conscious, of the analyst toward the patient. These may reflect the analyst's own unconscious conflicts and, if he is not constantly aware of this, may affect his understanding and therapeutic handling of the patient. In countertransference, the analyst has displaced onto the patient attitudes and feelings derived from earlier situations in his own life; the process is analogous to transference that involves the patient's similar reactions to the analyst. One of the cardinal purposes of the analyst's own analysis during his training is to make him aware of his own conflicts and their derivatives so that they do not distort his therapeutic work with patients. The analyst's continuing scrutiny of his own countertransference feelings frequently provides correct clues to the meaning of the patient's behavior, feelings, and thoughts and may facilitate more prompt perception of the patient's unconscious.

Interpretation: A form of intervention by the analyst, whose aim is to achieve therapeutic results by adding to the patient's knowledge of himself through making him aware of psychic content. In general, interpretations are dynamic or genetic in nature. Dynamic interpretations refer to psychic forces operating to produce a particular effect on mental life at any given time. Genetic interpretations are concerned with indicating or clarifying the connections between past mental states and present ones.

Insight: The subjective experiential knowledge acquired during psychoanalysis of previously unconscious pathogenic content and conflict. Analytic insight differs from other cognitive understanding in that it cannot occur without being preceded by dynamic changes leading to the weakening of resistances and the release of energies. These augment the autonomous ego functions that make insight possible. Among the more important autonomous ego functions involved are self-observation, synthesis, perception, memory and reality testing, control over regression and affective discharge, and integration.

Pseudo-insight may occur, in which there is apparent intellectual understanding of the forces involved, but instead of an integrative, energy-releasing function, the knowledge serves a libidinal or aggressive purpose with respect to the analyst, e.g., to please, to deceive, or to defeat him.

Supportive Therapy: Treatment in which the therapist intervenes directly in order to reintegrate the patient's impaired ego. This contrasts with analytic therapy, in which the therapist and patient work together, using the analysis of transference, in order to help the patient to diminish and control his neurotic reactions. Supportive therapy may include the use of psychoactive drugs, direct encouragement, expressions of positive regard by the therapist, or discussions of transference distortions in the context of present reality. For example, "You feel that I am against you but I am not. This clinic has suspended you because you broke the rules; we are not against you. These same rules apply to everyone being treated here."

Analytic Therapy: A form of treatment where past feelings, forbidden wishes, and the defenses associated with them are experienced in the interpersonal situation that develops between the patient and the therapist and in which these feelings are related to earlier life events. This expression of feelings, wishes, and defenses in the therapeutic situation is called the transference, and the process by which they are related to earlier life events is known as interpretation. The essence of analytic therapy is the patient's achievement of greater insight leading to mastery and progressive maturity of his affective responses through their subjective experience in the transference and its interpretation. In this way, analytic therapy can help the patient separate feelings appropriate to current life events from responses that are related to other processes. This can lead to a lessening of symptoms and an enrichment of the total personality.

Analytic therapy is a long and difficult process because many of the past feelings are unconscious and the patient often resists their expression and analysis. Successful analytic therapy requires that the patient simultaneously experience and observe his responses while, at the same time, collaborating with the analyst in the interpretive work. The development and interpretation of the transference distinguishes analytic from supportive therapy. Analytic therapy is usually used for neuroses but has been applied to borderline conditions and other, more serious disorders.

REFERENCES

Cohen, A. A Typology of Drug Addicts. Paper presented at the National Drug Abuse Conference. San Francisco, May 1977.

Greenacre, P. *Emotional Growth* (2 vols.). New York: Int. Univ. Press, 1971. vol. 1, pp. 225-248.

Jaffe, J. Verbal presentation given at National Academy of Sciences Meeting, McLean Hospital, Belmont, Massachusetts, November 1975a.

_____. Verbal presentation given at symposium on drug abuse problems, Aspen, Colorado, February 1975b.

Markovitz, E. On the nature of addiction to cigarettes. *J Amer Psychoanal Assoc*, 17:1076-1096, 1969.

Rogers, C. The process equation of psychotherapy. *Am J Psychiatry*, 15:27-45, 1961.

Rogers, C., Gendlin, E., Kiesler, D., and Truax, C., eds. *The Therapeutic Relationship and Its Impact: A Study of Psychotherapy With Schizophrenics.* Madison: U of Wisconsin Press, 1967.

Truax, C. Effective ingredients in psychotherapy: an approach to unraveling the patient-therapist interaction. *J Counseling Psychol*, 10:256-263, 1963.

Zinberg, N.E. Addiction and ego function. *Psychoanal Study Child*, 30:567-588, 1975.

BIBLIOGRAPHY

The following bibliography was compiled by computer search, as a convenient reference resource to encourage further research in the field of psychodynamics in drug dependence. It is offered in addition to the authors' references at the conclusion of each paper.

Black, F.W. Personality characteristics of Viet Nam veterans identified as heroin abusers. *American Journal of Psychiatry*, 132(7): 748-749, 1975.

Boyd, P. Heroin addiction in adolescents. *Journal of Psychosomatic Research*, 14:295-301, 1970.

Casselman, B.W. You cannot be a drug addict without really trying. *Diseases of the Nervous System*, 25:161-163, 1964.

Chatterji, N.N. Drug addiction and psychosis. *Samiksa*, 17(3):130-149, 1963.

Chein, I., Gerard, D.L., Lee, R.S, and Rosenfeld, E. Personality and addiction: A dynamic perspective. In: *The Road to H.* New York: Basic Books, 1964. pp. 227-250.

Chessick, R.D. The "pharmacogenic orgasm" in the drug addict. *Archives of General Psychiatry*, 3:545-556, 1960.

Coghlan, A.J., Gold, S.R., Dohrenwend, E.F., and Zimmerman, R.S. A psychobehavioral residential drug abuse program: A new adventure in adolescent psychiatry. *International Journal of the Addictions*, 8(5):767-777, 1973.

Copemann, C.D., and Shaw, P.L. The effect of therapeutic intervention on the assessment scores of narcotic addicts. *International Journal of the Addictions*, 10(5):921-926, 1975.

Coppolillo, H.P. Drug impediments to mothering behavior. *Addictive Diseases: An International Journal*, 2(1):201-208. 1975.

Crowley, R.M. Psychoanalytic literature on drug addiction and alcoholism. *Psychoanalytic Review*, 26:39-54, 1939.

Davis, W.N. The treatment of drug addiction: Some comparative observations. *British Journal of the Addictions*, 65:227-235, 1970.

DeLeon, G., Skodol, A., and Rosenthal, M.S. Phoenix House: Changes in psychopathological signs of resident drug addicts. *Archives of General Psychiatry*, 28:131-135, 1973.

Dole, V.P., and Nyswander, M.E. A medical treatment for diacetyl-morphine (heroin) addiction. *Journal of the American Medical Association*, 193(8):646-650, 1965.

Dole, V.P., and Nyswander, M.E. Methadone maintenance and its implication for theories of narcotic addiction. *Research Publications—Association for Research in Nervous and Mental Diseases*, 46:359-366, 1968.

Felix, R.H. Some comments on the psychopathology of drug addiction. *Mental Hygiene*, 23:567-582, 1939.

Felix, R.H. An appraisal of the personality types of the addict. *American Journal of Psychology*, 100:462-467, 1944.

Fenichel, O. Drug addiction. In: *The Psychoanalytic Theory of Neurosis*. New York: W. W. Norton, 1945. pp. 375-386.

Fisher, D., and DiMino, J.M. Case presentation of an alternative therapeutic approach for the borderline psychotic heroin addict: diphenylhydantoin. *British Journal of the Addictions*, 70(1):51-55, 1975.

Fram, D.H., and Hoffman, H.A. Family therapy in the treatment of the heroin addict. (Unpublished).

Fram, D.H., and Hoffman, H.A. Treatment of middle class heroin abusers: preliminary observations. *Medical Annals of the District of Columbia*, 41(5):301-303, 1972.

Frosch, W.A. Psychoanalytic evaluation of addiction and habituation. *Journal of the American Psychoanalytic Association*, 18:209-218, 1970.

Glatt, M.M. Psychotherapy of drug dependence: Some theoretical considerations. *British Journal of the Addictions*, 65:51-62, 1970.

Glover, E. On the aetiology of drug addiction. *International Journal of Psychoanalysis*, 13:298-328, 1932.

Guttman, O. The psychodynamics of a drug addict. *American Journal of Psychotherapy*, 19:653-665, 1965.

Hartmann, D. A study of drug-taking adolescents. *Psychoanalytic Study of the Child*, 24:384-398, 1969.

Hattersley, M. Heroin addiction and the psychiatric hospital. *Drug Forum*, 2(4):431-440, 1973.

Hendin, H. Students on heroin. *Journal of Nervous and Mental Disease*, 158(4):240-255, 1974.

Hoffman, M. Drug addiction and hypersexuality: Related modes of mastery. *Comprehensive Psychiatry*, 5(4):262-270, 1964.

Kaplan, E.H., and Wieder, H. Chapter X: "Treatment" and "Conclusion." In: *Drugs Don't Take People—People Take Drugs*, New York: Lyle Stewart, 1974.

Karp, E.G., Wurmser, L., and Savage, C. Therapeutic effects of methadone and LAAM (Two case reports), 1975 (Unpublished).

Kaufman, E. The psychodynamics of opiate dependence: A new look. *American Journal of Drug and Alcohol Abuse*, 1(3):349-370, 1974.

Kernberg, O. Borderline personality organization. *Journal of American Psychoanalytic Association*, 15(3):641-685, 1967.

Khantzian, E.J. Opiate addiction: A critique of theory and some implications for treatment. *American Journal of Psychotherapy*, 28(1):59-70, 1974.

Khantzian, E.J. Self selection and progression in drug dependence. *Psychiatry Digest*, pp. 19-22, 1975.

Khantzian, E.J., Mack, J.E., and Schatzberg, A.F. Heroin use as an attempt to cope: Clinical observations. *American Journal of Psychiatry*, 131(2):160-164, 1974.

Kohut, H. Preface to *Der Falsche Wag Zum Selbst, Studien Zur Drogankarriere*, by Jergen vom Scheidt, 1975.

Kolb, L. Types and characteristics: Drug addicts. *Mental Hygiene*, 9:300-313, 1925.

Kolb, L. Clinical contributions to drug addiction: The struggle for cure and the conscious reasons for relapse. *Journal of Nervous and Mental Disease*, 66:22-43, 1927.

Krystal, H. Withdrawal from drugs. *Psychosomatics*, 7:299-301, 1966.

Krystal, H. A review of *Drugs Don't Take People—People Take Drugs*. *The Psychoanalytic Quarterly*, 43:515-517, 1974.

Krystal, H., and Raskin, H.A. *Drug Dependence: Aspects of Ego Function*. Detroit: Wayne State University Press, 1970.

Laskowitz, D. The adolescent drug addict: An Adlerian view. *Journal of Individual Psychology*, 17:68-79, 1961.

Lief, V.F. Drug abuse: Models of treatment and their consequences. *International Pharmacopsychiatry*, 7(1-4):7-21, 1972.

Ling, W., Holmes, E.D., Post, G.R., and Litaker, M.B. A systematic psychiatric study of the heroin addicts. *National Conference on Methadone Treatment Proceedings*, 1:429-432, 1973.

Looney, M. The dreams of heroin addicts. *Social Work*, 17(6):23-28, 1972.

McKenna, G.J., Fisch, A., Levine, M.E., Patch, V.D., and Raynes, A.E. The use of methadone as a psychotropic agent. *National Conference on Methadone Treatment Proceedings*, 2:1317-1324, 1973.

Meerloo, J.A.M. Artificial ecstasy. *Journal of Nervous and Mental Disease*, 115:246-266, 1952.

Milkman, H., and Frosch, W.A. On the preferential abuse of heroin and amphetamine. *Journal of Nervous and Mental Disease*, 156(4):242-248, 1973.

Mott, J. The psychological basis of drug dependence: The intellectual and personality characteristics of opiate users. *British Journal of the Addictions*, 67:89-99, 1972.

Pittel, S.M. Psychological aspects of heroin and other drug dependence. *Journal of Psychedelic Drugs*, 1971, in press.

Proskauer, S., and Rolland, R.S. Youth who use drugs. Psychodynamic diagnosis and treatment planning. *Journal of the American Academy of Child Psychiatry*, 12(1):32-47, 1973.

Rado, S. The psychic effects of intoxicants: an attempt to evolve a psychoanalytical theory of morbid cravings. *International Journal of Psychoanalysis*, 7:396-413, 1926.

Rado, S. The psychoanalysis of pharmacothymia. *Psychoanalytic Quarterly*, 2:1-23, 1933.

Rado, S. Narcotic bondage: a general theory of the dependence on narcotic drugs. *American Journal of Psychiatry*, 114:165-170, 1957.

Raskin, H.A., Petty, T.A., and Warren, M. A suggested approach to the problem of narcotic addiction. *American Journal of Psychiatry*, 113:1089-1094, 1957.

Robbins, P.R. Depression and drug addiction. *Psychiatric Quarterly*, 48(3):374-386, 1974.

Robbins, P.R., and Nugent, III, J.F. Perceived consequences of addiction: A comparison between alcoholics and heroin-addicted patients. *Journal of Clinical Psychology*, 31(2):367-369, 1975.

Rosenfeld, H.A. The psychopathology of drug addiction and alcoholism: A critical review of the psychoanalytic literature (1964). In: *Psychotic States*. London: Hogarth Press, 1965.

Rosenfeld, H.A. On drug addiction (1960). In: *Psychotic States*. London: Hogarth Press, 1965.

Savitt, R.A. Clinical communications: Extramural psychoanalytic treatment of a case of narcotic addiction. *Journal of the American Psychoanalytic Association*, 2:494-502, 1954.

Savitt, R.A. Psychoanalytic studies on addiction: Ego structure in narcotic addiction. *Psychoanalytic Quarterly*, 32:43-57, 1963.

Schwartzman, J. The addict, abstinence, and the family. *American Journal of Psychiatry*, 132(2):154-157, 1975.

Senay, E.C., Dorus, W.W., and Meyer, E.P. Psychopathology in drug abusers, 1975 (Unpublished).

Sharoff, R.L. Character problems and their relationship to drug abuse. *American Journal of Psychoanalysis*, 29:186-193, 1969.

Singer, A. Mothering practices and heroin addiction. *American

Journal of Nursing, 74(1):77-82, 1974.

Szasz, T.S. The counterphobic mechanism in addiction. *Journal of the American Psychoanalytic Association*, 6:309-325, 1958.

Torda, C. Comments on the character structure and psychodynamic processes of heroin addicts. *Perceptual and Motor Skills*, 27(1): 143-146, 1968.

Vaillant, G.E. Sociopathy as a human process. *Archives of General Psychiatry*, 32:178-183, 1975.

Warren, W. The psychiatric approach—drug addiction. *Journal of the Royal College of General Practitioners*, 17:suppl. 2:2-8, 1969.

Wieder, H., and Kaplan, E.H. Drug use in adolescents: Psychodynamic meaning and pharmacogenic effect. *Psychoanalytic Study of the Child*, 24:399-431, 1969.

Wikler, A.A. A psychodynamic study of a patient during experimental self-regulated re-addiction to morphine. *Psychiatric Quarterly*, 26:270-293, 1952.

Wikler, A.A., and Rasor, R.W. Psychiatric aspects of drug addiction. *American Journal of Medicine*, 14:566-570, 1953.

Wishnie, H., and Cowan, R. Schematic techniques in therapy with addicts. *National Conference on Methadone Treatment Proceedings*, 2:1387-1393, 1973.

Woody, G.E., O'Brien, C.P., and Rickels, K. Depression and anxiety in heroin addicts: A placebo-controlled study of doxepin in combination with methadone. *American Journal of Psychiatry*, 132(4):447-450, 1975.

Wurmser, L. Why people take drugs: escape and search. *Maryland State Medical Journal*, Nov. 1970.

Wurmser, L. Drug abuse—nemesis of psychiatry. *American Scholar*, 41:393-407, 1972. Reprinted in *International Journal of Psychiatry* with critical evaluation and author's reply, 12:94-128, 1972.

Wurmser, L. Methadone and the craving for narcotics—observations of patients on methadone maintenance in psychotherapy. *Proceedings of the 4th National Methadone Conference*, 525-528, 1972.

Wurmser, L., Flowers, E., and Weldon, S., Methadone—discipline and revenge. *Proceedings of the 5th National Methadone Conference*, 1973.

Wurmser, L. Psychosocial aspects of drug abuse; Part 1: Etiological considerations. *Maryland State Medical Journal*, 22:78-82, 1973.

Wurmser, L. Psychosocial aspects of drug abuse; Part 2: Treatment and the role of the family physician. *Maryland State Medical Journal*, 22:99-101, 1973.

Wurmser, L. Personality disorders and drug dependency. In: *Personality Disorder Diagnosis and Management*, John R. Lion, ed., Baltimore: Williams & Wilkins, 113-142, 1974.

Wurmser, L. Psychoanaltyic considerations of the etiology of compulsive drug use. *Journal of the American Psychoanalytic Association*, 22(4):820-843, 1974.

Wurmser, L. *The Hidden Dimension: Psychopathology of Compulsive Drug Use*. New York: Jason Aronson, in press.

Wurmser, L., and Spiro, H.R. Factors in recognition and management of sociopathy and the addictions. In: *Modern Treatment*, 6:704-719, 1969.

Wurmser, L., Levin, L., and Lewis, A., Chronic paranoid and depressive symptoms in users of marihuana and LSD as observed in psychotherapy. *Proceedings of the 31st Annual Meeting of the Committee on Problems of Drug Dependence*. National Research Council, 1969.

Yorke, C. A critical review of some psychoanalytic literature on drug addiction. *British Journal of Medical Psychology*, 43:141-159, 1970.

Zimmering, P., Toolan, J., Safrin, M.S., and Wortis, S.B. Drug addiction in relation to problems of adolescence. *American Journal of Psychiatry*, 109:272-278, 1952.

Zinberg, N.E. Addiction and ego function. *Psychoanalytic Study of the Child*, 30:567-588, 1975.